Transfusion Science

Other books in the Biomedical Sciences Explained Series

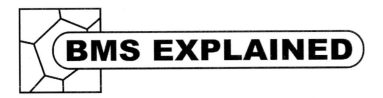

Transfusion Science

J. Overfield MPhil MSc FIBMS
Senior Lecturer in Biomedical Science, Department of Biological Sciences,
Manchester Metropolitan University, UK

M. Dawson BSc MSc PhD FIBMS
Senior Lecturer in Cell Biology and Immunology, Department of Biological Sciences,
Manchester Metropolitan University, UK

D. Hamer DMT FIBMS MHSM Cert HMS
Chief Biomedical Scientist, Transfusion Laboratory, Pathology Department,
Hope Hospital, Salford, UK

Series Editor:
C.J. Pallister PhD MSc FIBMS MIBiol CHSM
Principal Lecturer in Haematology, Department of Biological and Biomedical Sciences,
University of the West of England, Bristol, UK

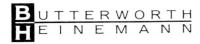

OXFORD AUCKLAND BOSTON JOHANNESBURG MELBOURNE NEW DELHI

Butterworth-Heinemann
Linacre House, Jordan Hill, Oxford OX2 8DP
225 Wildwood Avenue, Woburn, MA 01801-2041
A division of Reed Educational and Professional Publishing Ltd

℞ A member of the Reed Elsevier plc group

First published 1999

British Library Cataloguing in Publication Data
A catalogue record for this book is available from the British Library

Library of Congress Cataloguing in Publication Data
A catalogue record for this book is available from the Library of Congress

ISBN 0 7506 3415 4

Typeset by David Gregson Associates, Beccles, Suffolk
Printed and bound in Great Britain by Bath Press plc, Avon

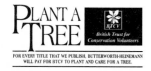

Contents

Preface

The science of transfusion is a constantly growing and changing subject. In recent years, new diseases have arisen which may be transmissible by blood and its components. Even as this book has been in progress, changes have occurred in society and our environment that future biomedical scientists in the transfusion world cannot ignore. Despite these impacts, the transfusion service strives to continue to provide safe products. In addition, much of the underlying learning basis for the student remains constant. For example, antigen and antibody structures and interactions, the mechanism of action of complement and autoimmune haemolysis are relatively well known. Changes are taking place in the field of transplantation and we have attempted to introduce students to the issues and requirements surrounding this important area as treatments continue to develop.

In this volume we hope to introduce medical and biomedical science students and scientists to basic principles in transfusion, whilst also increasing awareness of current issues and developments. We believe that this book will provide those who read it with a good basis on which to build their understanding of transfusion science.

We are grateful to Vin Sakalas at the Manchester Blood Centre for helpful advice on current issues with regard to blood products. Thanks also go to Chris Pallister and the staff at Butterworth-Heinemann for their advice and support and the co-authors would like to thank D. Hamer for the computer generated figures. Finally, we would like to thank our families for their patience.

J. Overfield, M. Dawson and D. Hamer

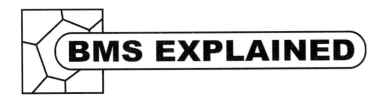

Series preface

The many disciplines that constitute the field of Biomedical Sciences have long provided excitement and challenge both for practitioners and for those who lead their education. This has never been truer than now as we ready ourselves to face the challenges of a new millennium. The exponential growth in biomedical enquiry and knowledge seen in recent years has been mirrored in the education and training of biomedical scientists. The burgeoning of modular BSc (Hons) Biomedical Sciences degrees and the adoption of graduate-only entry by the Institute of Biomedical Sciences and the Council for Professions Supplementary to Medicine have been important drivers of change.

The broad range of subject matter encompassed by the Biomedical Sciences has led to the design of modular BSc (Hons) Biomedical Sciences degrees that facilitate wider undergraduate choice and permit some degree of specialization. There is a much greater emphasis on self-directed learning and understanding of learning outcomes than hitherto.

Against this background, the large, expensive standard texts designed for single subject specialization over the duration of the degree and beyond, are much less useful for the modern student of biomedical sciences. Instead, there is a clear need for a series of short, affordable, introductory texts, which assume little prior knowledge and which are written in an accessible style. The *Biomedical Sciences Explained* series is specifically designed to meet this need.

Each book in the series is designed to meet the needs of a level 1 or 2 student and will have the following distinctive features:

- written by experienced academics in the biomedical sciences in a student-friendly and accessible style, with the trend towards student-centred and life-long learning firmly in mind;
- each chapter opens with a set of defined learning objectives and closes with self-assessment questions which check that the learning objectives have been met;
- aids to understanding such as potted histories of important scientists, descriptions of seminal experiments and background information appear as sideboxes;
- extensively illustrated with line diagrams, charts and tables wherever appropriate;
- use of unnecessary jargon is avoided. New terms are explained, either in the text or sideboxes;
- written in an explanatory rather than a didactic style, emphasizing conceptual understanding rather than rote learning.

I sincerely hope that you find these books as helpful in your studies as they have been designed to be. Good luck and have fun!

C. J. Pallister

To Michael, Catherine, Emma, Vicki, Julia, Karen, David and Holly-Jayne

and

to Peter Howell of the Manchester Blood Centre, in recognition of his invaluable
contribution to teaching in transfusion science

Chapter 1
The immune system

Learning objectives

After studying this chapter you should confidently be able to:

Discuss the differences between non-specific and specific immune defences.

Outline the roles of complement, interferons and cytokines in the non-specific defences.

Describe the cells of the non-specific defences and outline their roles.

Describe the major features of inflammation and the acute phase response.

Discuss the differences between humoral and cell-mediated immunity.

Define the terms immunogen, antigen, epitope and hapten.

Discuss the roles of B and T lymphocytes in specific immune responses.

The study of immunology in modern times dates from the eighteenth century when Edward Jenner investigated the popular belief that infection with cowpox could protect against the often lethal smallpox virus. After years of investigation, he showed that he could fully protect individuals from smallpox by deliberately inoculating them with cowpox material. His results were published in 1798 in a document entitled '*An inquiry into the causes and effects of the Variolae Vaccinae, a disease discovered in some of the Western Counties of England particularly Gloucestershire and known by the name of the Cowpox*'. Since then, immunologists have made astonishing progress in determining how the immune system protects individuals from infectious disease. In addition, scientists have also been able to make use of products of the immune system in many different ways. Antibodies, for example, are used for developing highly sensitive assays and cytokines are used therapeutically. Much of this progress has been made in the last 40 years, although antibodies have been recognized for much longer than that.

The immune system

The bodies of multicellular animals are constantly threatened by the multitude of micro-organisms that exist outside them. Many of these micro-organisms are potentially pathogenic, that is, they can cause disease. They may cause disease in a number of ways: for example, bacteria can produce toxins, while viruses enter living cells and may eventually lyse them. Parasites may subvert the normal physiological mechanisms in many different ways (e.g. *Plasmodium*, the malarial parasite, lyses red cells, causes a kidney disease called glomerulonephritis and may cause damage to small blood vessels).

All multicellular animals have defence mechanisms both to keep out potentially harmful micro-organisms and to remove them from the body if they enter. The set of defence mechanisms is known as the **immune system.**

The human immune system is essentially the same as the immune system of other mammals and similar to that of other higher vertebrates. This immune system is able to distinguish between the cells and macromolecules that make up the body and those that do not. In other words, the immune system is able to distinguish between **self** and **non-self**. It is essential that transfusion science students understand how the immune system works because it is this ability to distinguish self from non-self which underlies the reasons why donated blood should match the blood of the recipient and why the best chance of survival following a transplant occurs when the donated organ has been 'matched' to the recipient through the process known as **tissue typing**. The consequences of mismatched transfusions are discussed in Chapter 7. Immunological components other than blood may be transfused or may be used in transfusion science methodology, for example antibodies (Chapter 2) and complement (Chapter 3).

Two types of immune defence

Immunological defences are usually classified into two kinds, depending on what exactly is being recognized. For example, some defences are **non-specific** and these are targeted at any material which is foreign to the body, including substances such as wood splinters, as well as micro-organisms. This is one of the reasons why materials used in medical prostheses, especially those fitted internally like artificial hip joints, have to be thoroughly tested before use. If unsuitable, they may trigger the body's defence mechanisms and induce an unacceptable inflammatory reaction.

As well as non-specific defences there is a series of **specific** immune defences in which cells and macromolecules are able to recognize not only individual micro-organisms but also the particular proteins or glycoproteins which make up that micro-organism. The specific immune system is extremely important for maintaining health because, once activated, it can result in **immunity** to a micro-organism. Finally, non-specific defences are available immediately, as soon as an organism enters the body, and they constitute a first line of defence. A specific immune response, on the other hand, may take several days to produce its effect. In transfusion, this may explain why a haemolytic reaction to foreign red blood cells may sometimes occur several days after the transfusion has taken place. It is important to remember, though, that the distinctions between non-specific and specific immunological defences can become blurred because there are so many interactions between the two. For example, non-specific cells such as macrophages are often required to initiate specific immunity and, once activated, the products of this system bring about removal of micro-organisms, for the most part, by stimulating the non-specific defences.

Non-specific defences

A list of some of the important non-specific defences is given in Table 1.1. Some of these defences that are relevant to transfusion science are discussed below.

Complement

Complement is the name given to a set of proteins found in fresh plasma which has a variety of important immunological roles. These include causing lysis of micro-organisms and stimulating phagocytosis and inflammation. Complement proteins are present

Table 1.1 *The major non-specific immunological defences*

Defence	Example
Structural barriers	Skin, mucosal membranes
Acidity	Lactic acid in sweat, HCl in stomach
Proteins	Complement, lysozyme, interferons
Phagocytic cells	Monocytes, macrophages, neutrophilic polymorphonuclear leukocytes (neutrophils), eosinophilic polymorphonuclear leukocytes (eosinophils)
Non-phagocytic cells	Natural killer (NK) cells, basophilic polymorphonuclear leukocytes (basophils)
Physiological responses	Inflammation, the acute phase response

People who have an active viral infection are commonly resistant to infection with another virus, a phenomenon known as viral 'interference' which was first described by Jenner in 1804. An interferon is now defined as a protein which 'exerts non-specific antiviral activity at least in homologous cells through cellular metabolic processes involving synthesis of both RNA and protein' (Interferon Nomenclature Committee, 1980).

Interest in interferons was greatly enhanced in the 1970s when it was shown that interferon α could cause regression of some animal tumours and could inhibit the growth of cultured cancer cells. Since then, interferons have been tested extensively in cancer patients but success has been limited to a few types of cancer. Interferons are now being used in the treatment of other diseases, including multiple sclerosis.

A number of cytokines are now used therapeutically in treating several diseases. One of the first to be tested was interleukin 2 (IL-2), which has been used to treat renal cancer and melanoma. G-CSF (granulocyte-colony stimulating factor) has been used to stimulate the growth of bone marrow after depletion with cytotoxic drugs for the treatment of leukaemia (see Chapter 11). Other cytokines have been implicated in disease processes; for example, there is evidence for the involvement of TNF-α in the development of septic shock and cerebral malaria. In such cases cytokine antagonists, such as antibodies to TNF, may be useful in treatment.

in an inactive form in plasma but they may become activated by the micro-organism itself (the alternative pathway) or by antibodies bound to a micro-organism (the classical pathway). This is discussed in detail in Chapter 3. Complement can also be activated by other proteins such as C-reactive protein (CRP) and mannan-binding lectin (MBL) which are produced early in an infection by cells in the liver.

Interferons

Interferons (IFNs) are families of inducible secretory proteins produced by eukaryotic cells in response to viral infection and other stimuli. They were first discovered by Isaacs and Lindenmann in 1957 who showed that cultured fragments of chick embryo chorioallantoic membrane deliberately infected with influenza virus secreted a substance into the culture medium which could interfere with viral replication. Interferons are not directly antiviral but act to prevent viral infection by inducing healthy cells to produce enzymes which inhibit replication of viral nucleic acid and production of viral protein.

There are three major families of interferons: α, β and γ. Interferons α and β are both produced by cells which have been infected with a virus. Interferon γ, which was discovered by Wheelock in 1965, is produced by cells of the specific immune system in response to any agent, whether a bacterium, virus or foreign protein, which stimulates that system. Interferons are examples of a very broad family of proteins known as **cytokines**. Since this term will be used frequently in discussing the immune system and transfusion, this is probably a good point at which to define it.

Cytokines

Cytokines are proteins secreted by cells that bind to cell surface receptors on other cells and induce particular activities in them. They therefore act as molecules of communication between cells. Cytokines act at very low concentrations (e.g. 10^{-10} M) and will stimulate only those cells that have the appropriate receptors. Cytokines may act, for example, to stimulate the growth or differentiation of cells or may promote the synthesis of proteins by particular cells. Many cytokines are involved in the immune response, and several will be mentioned by the end of this chapter. Several cytokines are now used therapeutically. In bone marrow transplantation, for example, cytokines may be used to stimulate the growth of engrafted tissue. Cytokines may also have pathological consequences in transfusion. For example, cytokines may 'leak' from white blood cells in donor blood and can cause damage to tissues of the recipient (see Chapter 10).

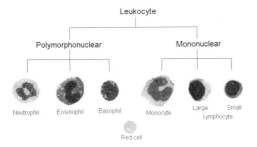

Figure 1.1 *The leukocytes – a red blood cell is also shown for comparison*

Cells of the non-specific defences

All of the white blood cells have a role in the immune system though not all of them are phagocytes. The white blood cells are classified into two groups, according to the shape of the nucleus: **polymorphonuclear leukocytes (PMN)** have a nucleus which is lobed and **mononuclear leukocytes (MN)** have a nucleus which is more rounded (see Figure 1.1).

Polymorphonuclear leukocytes

Approximately 70% of blood leukocytes are polymorphonuclear. They have a granular cytoplasm and for this reason are also known as **granulocytes**. Three types are found in the blood: the **neutrophil**, the **basophil** and the **eosinophil**, each with distinct functions in defending the body from potential pathogens.

The neutrophil

The most abundant and most easily recognized leukocyte is the neutrophil, which makes up about 65% of the total blood leukocytes in adults. It has a highly lobed nucleus, typically with between three and five lobes. The neutrophil is a phagocytic cell and is highly efficient at ingesting bacteria, especially if they are coated with antibody or complement. Neutrophils are often called **inflammatory cells** because they are always the first cells to arrive at a site of inflammation.

Neutrophils are short-lived cells. They are produced in the bone marrow and released into the blood, where they circulate for a mere 24 hours. After this time the cell dies and is removed by other phagocytic cells, chiefly monocytes in the blood and macrophages in the spleen. The number of blood neutrophils increases within a few hours of an infection becoming established because the bone marrow is stimulated, by cytokines, to release neutrophil reserves.

Neutrophils which ingest living bacteria, whether antibody-coated or not, take the bacteria into the cytoplasm in phagocytic vacuoles. Within the cell there are several mechanisms for killing bacteria:

- Primary lysosomes or granules containing hydrolytic enzymes capable of breaking down most biological macromolecules fuse with the phagocytic vacuoles and release these enzymes on to the bacterium.
- Accompanying the uptake of bacteria is a burst of respiration which results in the production of hydrogen peroxide. Hydrogen peroxide is then converted to hypochlorite in the presence of chloride ions and the enzyme myeloperoxidase. Both hydrogen peroxide and hypochlorite have considerable antibacterial properties.
- The cytoplasm of the neutrophil also contains small molecular weight proteins, known as defensins, which attack the bacterial membrane, rendering it permeable.
- Although neutrophils are able to ingest uncoated bacteria, binding to bacteria that have been coated with antibody and/or complement actually stimulates uptake and the various bactericidal mechanisms. The promotion of phagocytosis in this way is known as **opsonization.**

The basophil

Basophils make up only a small percentage of the blood leukocytes – generally less than 1%. The term basophil refers to the fact that the granules in the cytoplasm take up basic stains such as toluidine blue. Basophils have a bilobed nucleus and very prominent cytoplasmic granules which contain a number of pharmacologically active chemicals. These include histamine, which dilates blood vessels and increases blood vessel permeability, heparin, which inhibits blood clotting, chemotactic factors which attract neutrophils and eosinophils, and a protease which degrades the basement membrane of blood vessels.

Although the basophil is found in the blood, there is a similar type of cell found in solid tissues. This cell is the **mast cell** and it has cytoplasmic granules with contents similar to those found in the basophil, although its precise relationship to the basophil is uncertain. The mast cell is found in many solid tissues including the skin, the mucosal membranes and epithelia of the respiratory, genitourinary and gastrointestinal tracts, and in the connective tissue of a variety of internal organs. The role of mast cells and basophils is to trigger the process of inflammation, which can be stimulated by antibodies (see Chapter 2).

The eosinophil

Eosinophils usually make up less than 2% of the blood leukocytes. Like the basophils, they have a highly granular cytoplasm. Unlike the basophils, however, the granules in this case contain highly basic proteins which readily take up acidic stains such as eosin. Although eosinophils have been shown to be phagocytic cells, this role is probably a minor one. The major role of the eosinophil is to assist in the elimination of multicellular parasites such as tapeworms and nematodes. Eosinophils first bind to the surface of the worm, often via antibody, and then expel the granular proteins on to the worm surface. The number of eosinophils in the blood is also increased in patients suffering from certain types of allergy, including hay fever and allergic asthma.

Mononuclear leukocytes

While this group constitutes only 30% of the blood leukocytes it contains some of the most important cells in the immune response. Two of these, the **monocytes** and the **large granular lymphocytes** (LGL), are non-specific cells. The last group, **the small lymphocytes,** will dominate the remainder of this chapter, since they are responsible for the specific immune response.

Monocytes

Monocytes comprise approximately 5% of the blood leukocytes. They have a characteristic indented, often horseshoe-shaped, nucleus and a granular cytoplasm (see Figure 1.1). Monocytes in the blood may be regarded as cells 'in transit'. They are produced in the bone marrow, they circulate in the blood for 8 hours and then migrate to the solid tissues where they develop into **macrophages**. Macrophages may be 'fixed' in tissues or they may wander in an amoeboid fashion throughout the tissues (see Table 1.2). Organs that have an especially high content of macrophages include the spleen, the lungs, the liver, the lymph nodes and the tonsils. Monocytes and macrophages, wherever located, form the **mononuclear phagocytic system,** otherwise known as the **reticuloendothelial system,** which clears foreign and senescent material from tissues by phagocytosis. Like the neutrophils, these cells bind readily to complement- and antibody-coated material, favouring opsonization. Macrophages in particular are highly active phagocytes with a range of killing mechanisms similar to the neutrophil.

Macrophages are activated by several cytokines, especially interferon γ (IFN-γ) which is produced by some types of small

Table 1.2   *The mononuclear phagocytic system (reticuloendothelial system)*

Fixed tissue macrophages	Mobile macrophages
Kupffer cells (liver)	Spleen
Alveolar macrophages (lungs)	Lymph nodes
Histiocytes (connective tissue)	Tonsils
Mesangial cells (kidney)	
Microglial cells (brain)	

When cells are 'killed' through a toxic environmental agent, or perhaps through lack of oxygen to the tissue (anoxia), or loss of blood supply (ischaemia), they die through a process known as necrosis. Death by necrosis is somewhat 'messy' because the cell contents leak out into the surrounding tissue and can stimulate inflammation. In contrast, the vast majority of cell death is brought about by a much 'neater' method in which death is programmed. Apoptosis involves rapid fragmentation of cellular DNA and the breaking up of the cell into membrane-bound apoptotic bodies which are eventually phagocytosed. The genetic control of this system is now being unravelled and may prove useful in the treatment of cancer.

lymphocytes. In addition, when stimulated they produce a range of cytokines, including interleukins 1 (IL-1), 6 (IL-6) and 8 (IL-8) and tumour necrosis factor (TNF) α. Secretion of these cytokines is stimulated following phagocytosis, especially of micro-organisms. Interleukins 1 and 6 together with TNF-α are known to be responsible for bringing about the non-specific response known as the **acute phase response**, an early response to infection. IL-8 is a cytokine which is known to attract neutrophils.

As well as clearing foreign material from the body, macrophages are also important for removing old and dying cells. Neutrophils, for example, live for only 24 hours in the body. Their death is programmed genetically and self-destruction, a process known as **apoptosis**, occurs. Macrophages are able to detect cells undergoing apoptosis and remove them. In the spleen, macrophages remove old and worn-out (effete) red blood cells from the circulation. Complement is also involved in this process.

Finally, monocytes and macrophages are also involved in triggering the specific immune system. They 'process' foreign material in such a way that it can be recognized by small lymphocytes. In this respect they are known as **antigen-presenting cells (APC)**.

Large granular lymphocytes

Large granular lymphocytes (LGL) make up between 5 and 10% of the blood leukocytes. These cells have a rounded nucleus and a granular cytoplasm (see Figure 1.1). They represent a mixed population of cells in terms of function. Some LGL act as natural killer (NK) cells. These cells have a role in antiviral immunity because they kill cells that have been infected with a virus. Although they do not recognize a particular virus, they help to prevent viral replication. NK cells are not phagocytic but kill by releasing proteins on to the target cell which perforate the cell membrane and may induce apoptosis of the infected cell. NK cells are probably also important in destroying cancer cells as they arise in the body.

Some LGL are also known to be able to kill target cells coated with antibody, a function which is discussed in Chapter 2.

Non-specific responses to tissue damage and infection

A micro-organism or some other foreign material which breaches the external barriers that generally keep such items out (e.g. skin, mucosal membranes) is subject to attack by various proteins and cells. This attack takes place in two important immunological responses known as **inflammation** and the **acute phase response**:

- **Inflammation** is a rapid and local response, initially to tissue damage, which may later become a chronic response if an infection persists at the site of damage. It is characterized by reddening, swelling, heat and pain at the damaged site. Anyone who has ever scratched their skin or had a blister caused by badly fitting shoes will be familiar with these symptoms. Inflammation is initiated by the release of histamine from mast cells in the damaged area. Histamine stimulates dilation of blood vessels, contributing to the reddening and local 'heat'. The blood vessels become 'leaky' so that plasma flows out into the damaged tissue. Neutrophils may also move across the blood vessel walls, between the lining endothelial cells. The process of inflammation serves to dilute out any harmful substance which may have entered damaged tissue and to initiate its removal by promoting the influx of neutrophils into the inflamed site.

- **The acute phase response** occurs within hours of exposure to micro-organisms, though it may also be induced following extensive tissue damage such as burns to the skin. This response may also occur as the result of a transfusion reaction. The acute phase response is a systemic (whole body) response involving several organ systems and is brought about by cytokines released by monocytes and macrophages. These cells release IL-1, IL-6 and TNF-α, which together induce a number of effects (see Table 1.3). There are notable changes in the composition of the blood during an acute phase response, including an increase in neutrophils and increases in a number of defence proteins known as the **acute phase proteins**. One of the most well known of these proteins is C-reactive protein (CRP). The plasma concentration of CRP prior to an acute phase response is so low as to be barely measurable; thereafter its synthesis increases 100- to 1000-fold. It is a protein which can bind to certain bacteria and cause their destruction by activating complement.

The effects of the acute phase response are (mostly) beneficial, even if they may not appear to be (e.g. fever, drowsiness). However, many effects of the acute phase response have the potential to be harmful if an infection is prolonged. In the event of an acute phase response following a transfusion reaction, the effects are inappropriate since no infectious agent is present, and the symptoms of the acute phase response may increase the discomfort for the patient.

Inflammation and the acute phase response are very much interlinked, as indeed are all immunological responses. A chronic infection will result in a prolonged acute phase response and the long-term production of molecules which also stimulate inflammation.

The specific immune response

The specific immune response allows the development of true 'immunity' to an infectious agent. Since true immunity can only

Table 1.3 *Physiological changes during an acute phase response*

Physiological change	Biological significance
Fever	Increase in body temperature may inhibit the growth of bacteria and favour the development of specific immunity
Increased drowsiness	Possibly conserving energy
Loss of appetite	People often lose weight during an infectious illness even though they have a higher nutritional requirement because of the increased protein synthesis taking place. During chronic infection this weight loss may be highly significant.
Increase in protein content in the blood	This represents increases in the acute phase proteins which are synthesized in the liver
Increased amino acid content of blood	These amino acids are derived from the breakdown of muscle protein. The amino acids are used by the liver to synthesize the acute phase proteins
Increased number of neutrophils in the blood	These are released from reserves in the bone marrow
Decreased blood zinc and iron levels	Removal inhibits the growth of bacteria
Loss of muscle tissue	The liver is supplied with amino acids to support the production of acute phase proteins. These amino acids are provided by the proteolytic breakdown of muscle tissue. This contributes to the severe 'wasting' of muscles (a condition known as cachexia) that can occur in chronic infections

develop after exposure to the micro-organism (or a 'harmless' vaccine created from the micro-organism), the response is often called '**acquired**'. For example, an individual who has had measles is very unlikely to get that disease again, even though they may be exposed to the virus several times in their lifetime.

During the course of an infection such as measles, two types of specific immunity are activated. These are **humoral immunity** and **cell-mediated immunity**.

Humoral immunity involves the production of **antibodies**. These are glycoproteins found in the plasma, lymph and body secretions such as saliva, tears, mucus and milk. Antibodies are specific to the micro-organism that induced them (the **immunogen**). Once produced, they bind to the microbe and mark it out for destruction (see

Chapter 2). Antibodies are produced by cells in lymphoid tissues. They are released into the lymph and eventually reach the blood.

Cell-mediated immunity (CMI) involves the destruction of micro-organisms by direct and indirect means. First, there is the production of **cytotoxic cells** capable of killing any cell infected with the micro-organism that induced them. Cytotoxic cells are especially important in antiviral immunity because viruses are obligate parasites which 'hide' within the cells they infect. Destroying infected cells inhibits the virus from replicating while antibody can 'mop-up' any virus released from dead cells. Cytotoxic cells are specific, which means they will recognize and kill cells only if they recognize the virus that is infecting them. Thus cytotoxic cells raised by a measles infection will not kill cells infected with rubella virus and vice versa.

A second type of killing in CMI is indirect and is mediated by cells of the specific response releasing cytokines which encourage the phagocytes, especially macrophages, to kill the micro-organism.

The important features to remember about specific immunity are as follows:

- Specific immunity is only induced towards the agent which stimulated it (i.e. the immunogen).
- On second contact with the immunogen, the specific immune response is mobilized more rapidly than on first contact. It is this rapid response which prevents development of the disease in an immune individual because antibodies and cytotoxic cells can attack the micro-organism before it causes clinical symptoms. This ability to produce a quicker response on second contact with an immunogen is known as **immunological memory**.

Immunogens

Anything which stimulates a specific immune response is called an immunogen (see Table 1.4). Micro-organisms and foreign cells, e.g. red blood cells, are powerful immunogens. This is because they are composed of immunogenic macromolecules such as proteins and glycoproteins. It has been estimated that a protein must have a molecular weight of at least 5000 daltons (Da) to be immunogenic and, generally speaking, the larger the protein, the

Table 1.4 *Major groups of immunogens*

Immunogen	*Example*
Micro-organisms	Bacteria, viruses, protozoa, multicellular parasites, fungi
Foreign cells	Red blood cells, transplants
Macromolecules	Proteins, glycoproteins, lipoproteins, complex polysaccharides, nucleic acids

more immunogenic it will be, so long as it is foreign to the body. Thus the protein hormone pig insulin, with a molecular weight of 5172 Da, is weakly immunogenic in humans.

Some more definitions

At this stage, it would be useful to provide some definitions related to immunogens and precisely what it is about immunogens that the immune system recognizes.

Antigen

While the term immunogen is used to describe something which stimulates the specific immune response, the term antigen is used to describe something which reacts with the products of the immune response. Thus, an antigen may be part of a protein, such as a small polypeptide, which by itself is too small to stimulate specific immunity but, once an immune response has been initiated, is able to combine with the products of that immune response. The term 'antigen' is often used when referring to antibodies reacting with molecules *in vitro*, for example during an immunoassay such as a radioimmunoassay or in the agglutination tests that are used in the transfusion laboratory.

Epitope

The epitope is the small part of the immunogen that is recognized by the cells of the specific immune system. It is also that part of the antigen to which an antibody can bind. The epitopes on a protein consist of regions of between five and seven amino acids in length, and an immunogenic protein may have a number of epitopes that are recognized as 'foreign'.

Hapten

Some relatively small molecules, such as dinitrophenol, are far too small to stimulate an immune response when administered as the free molecule. However, such small molecules, known as haptens, can be covalently attached to an immunogenic protein, known as a carrier, to form a hapten–carrier complex. When such complexes are administered to animals by injection, they stimulate the production of antibodies not only to the protein carrier but also to the hapten. This implies that the immune system has cells capable of recognizing these small molecules as foreign, but is unable to respond until these haptens are presented to the immune system in the right way (almost as an additional epitope on the carrier protein). Some drugs induce immune haemolytic anaemias when they bind to proteins on red cell membranes and act as haptens, inducing antibody production against them.

Relative importance of humoral and cell-mediated immunity

Most immunogens stimulate both humoral and cell-mediated immunity. However, as a general rule, humoral immunity is more important in combating micro-organisms which are extracellular parasites, i.e. they live outside the cells of the host. Since antibody is found in the body fluids, including blood and lymph, there will not be a problem concerning access of the antibody to the immunogen. In contrast, CMI is involved with immunity to parasites which live inside cells; for example, all viruses are absolutely dependent on cells for their replication. Certain bacteria, too, habitually live within the cells of the host. Examples of intracellular bacteria include *Mycobacterium tuberculosis* and *Listeria monocytogenes*. In this case, antibodies have no access to the parasites and CMI is more significant.

Specific immune responses are obviously beneficial and they are the chief defences against invasion by micro-organisms. There are, however, occasions when they are definitely unwanted. Humoral immunity, for example, is responsible for a range of allergic reactions including hay fever and allergic asthma. Antibodies are responsible for blood transfusion reactions, haemolytic anaemias and some occupational diseases such as Farmer's lung. Cell-mediated immunity is the cause of allergic contact dermatitis and is the main reason for the rejection of transplanted tissue. CMI is also responsible for the **graft versus host** reaction which may be a fatal consequence of bone marrow transplantation (see Chapter 11).

> The ability of the immune system to make antibodies against a range of molecules which are not in themselves immunogenic has been utilized by industry as well as in biological and biomedical research. For example, antibodies against steroid hormones are routinely used to measure the concentration of these hormones in plasma. They can also be used to detect anabolic steroids and their metabolites in the urine of athletes. Antibodies can be used to detect and treat overdoses of digoxin in patients taking the drug to treat cardiac arrhythmias.

Cells of the specific immune response

The small lymphocyte is responsible for the specific immune response, a fact which was only proven in the 1960s. This cell (see Figure 1.1) is found in blood where it makes up approximately 20% of the leukocytes. Far more small lymphocytes, however, are found outside the blood, in the lymphoid tissues. **Primary lymphoid tissues**, such as the **thymus**, are important sites of maturation for small lymphocytes, whereas the **secondary lymphoid tissues**, such as the spleen, the lymph nodes, the tonsils and mucosa-associated lymphoid tissue (MALT), are the sites of activity of the mature small lymphocytes and are also the places where antibody-producing cells are found.

Development of small lymphocytes

The population of small lymphocytes is one of the most heterogeneous in the body, despite the fact that all small lymphocytes have a very similar appearance. However, it is possible to classify them into two major groups depending initially on where they develop, and into at least three major groups depending on what they do.

Cells which give rise to small lymphocytes are first produced in the bone marrow, following successive divisions of the **lymphoid stem cells**. During foetal development some of these immature lymphocytes leave the bone marrow and enter the thymus, a bilobed gland found in the upper anterior midline of the chest, where they mature. Lymphocytes that mature in the thymus are known as **thymus-dependent** or **T lymphocytes**. Two different types of mature T lymphocyte are produced in the thymus: the **helper T lymphocytes** (T_H) and the **cytotoxic precursor T lymphocytes** (T_C). The function of these cells is discussed below. In mammals, the second group of small lymphocytes completes its development within the bone marrow. When mature, these cells are known as **B lymphocytes**.

When mature, B and T lymphocytes leave the primary lymphoid tissues and can be found in the blood and secondary lymphoid tissues. Small lymphocytes are constantly moving between the blood and the lymphoid compartments, a process known as **recirculation**. Small lymphocytes move across the endothelial cells of the blood vessels that supply the lymphoid tissues and enter the lymphatic system. They emerge from lymphoid tissue with the efferent lymph, a fluid that eventually enters the blood supply at the point where the major lymphatic vessel, the thoracic duct, joins up with the left subclavian vein in the neck. Each small lymphocyte can only respond to a single epitope and recirculation is essential to ensure that the specific small lymphocytes come into contact with immunogens bearing the epitopes to which they are specific.

Role of T and B lymphocytes

B lymphocytes are responsible for humoral immunity. When stimulated they give rise to antibody-producing cells. T_C cells are the precursors of the cytotoxic cells. When stimulated they give rise to cytotoxic T lymphocytes (CTL) which are predominantly involved in killing virus-infected cells. T_H are regulatory cells. When stimulated they release an array of cytokines that influence all aspects of the immune response.

Distinguishing T and B lymphocytes

It is not possible to distinguish between T and B lymphocytes or between T_H and T_C in a conventional blood smear. In order to tell

The role of the thymus was established in the 1960s when it was shown that removing the thymus from a neonatal mouse (neonatal thymectomy) had profound effects on the immune response: blood lymphocyte levels were greatly reduced, the spleen and lymph nodes were underdeveloped, cell-mediated immunity was impaired and the animals were very prone to viral infections. Antibody levels were reduced but not absent.

Birds have a second primary lymphoid organ called the Bursa of Fabricius. This organ is not present in mammals. Removing the Bursa of Fabricius from chick embryos was shown to affect humoral immunity but left cell-mediated immunity intact. Bursectomized birds are prone to bacterial, but not viral, infections and antibodies are not found in the plasma. B lymphocytes were therefore named as such because they are **bursa-dependent** in birds. B lymphocytes are responsible for antibody production. In mammals, the 'B' does not stand for bone marrow derived, since both B and T cells originate in the bone marrow. In fact, B cells in mammals are **bursa equivalent cells** because they have the same role in humoral immunity as the bursa-dependent cells in birds.

them apart it is necessary to stain for particular protein markers on the membranes of the individual cells. This can be achieved using the technique of **immunofluorescence**, using an antibody to the marker in question which has been chemically labelled with a fluorochrome (a molecule that will fluoresce when irradiated with light of a shorter wavelength). B lymphocytes have antibodies in their membranes. The cells can be 'stained' with a fluorescent anti-antibody. All mature T lymphocytes have a molecule known as CD3 which is associated with the T-cell receptor and can be detected with a fluorescent anti-CD3. T_H cells have the protein CD4 in their membranes, whereas T_C cells have CD8, and therefore these cells can be distinguished with the appropriate antibody.

Specificity of small lymphocytes

All small lymphocytes are specific for a single epitope on an individual immunogen. This means that they will only respond to that epitope and no other. The specificity lies in the fact that each of these cells has membrane-bound proteins which act as receptors for an individual epitope. The receptors on B lymphocytes are membrane-bound antibodies, each of which has two epitope-binding sites. The T-cell receptor (TCR) is composed of two single polypeptide chains with a single binding site. All the receptors on a single small lymphocyte, be it a T cell or a B cell, have the same specificity.

When an epitope binds to a receptor on a small lymphocyte, in the appropriate manner, the small lymphocyte starts to divide many times and forms a clone of identical cells, all with the same specificity (Figure 1.2), greatly increasing the number of cells bearing that particular receptor. Most of the cells in this clone then differentiate, under the influence of a number of cytokines, into 'effector' cells. Some cells in the clone do not differentiate but remain at this stage until the next exposure to the same immunogen.

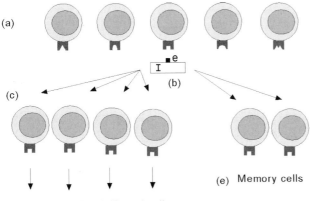

(a)

(b)

(c)

(d) Differentiation into 'effector' cells

(e) Memory cells

Figure 1.2 *Clonal selection. (a) Small lymphocytes are specific for an epitope because they each have cell surface receptors for an individual epitope. (b) When a cell binds the right epitope (e) on the surface of an immunogen (I), this cell is stimulated to proliferate to form a clone of identical cells (c). Some of the cells in this clone differentiate into effector cells (d) while others remain as memory cells (e)*

These cells are the **memory cells.** The quicker response shown on second contact with an immunogen is, at least in part, due to having more of the 'right' sort of cells available.

Activation of B lymphocytes

B lymphocytes have receptors which bind 'native' epitope. This means that they can be stimulated directly by the epitope as it occurs on the immunogen. When B lymphocytes bind the epitope, they proliferate and develop into plasma cells (see Figure 1.3). Plasma cells are fully differentiated antibody-secreting cells. Plasma cells do not recirculate but 'home' to lymphoid tissues where they continue to secrete antibody until they die (a matter of weeks). The antibody they produce is homogeneous and has the same specificity as the B-cell receptor antibodies, ensuring that only the required antibody is produced. In fact, each B cell is only capable of producing antibody of one specificity and this is determined during the development of the B cell in the bone marrow. Antibody secreted by plasma cells in lymphoid tissues appears first in the lymph and then in the blood.

Cytokine involvement

The proliferation of B lymphocytes and their differentiation into plasma cells requires cytokines which are produced by the T_H cells. Certain cytokines favour the production of antibodies of different classes. For example, interleukin 4 (IL-4) promotes the production of IgE. This requirement for T cells in the production of antibody is seen in the response to most immunogens, which are often referred to as 'T-dependent'. This also explains the poor antibody production in mice that have had their thymus surgically removed in the first week of life.

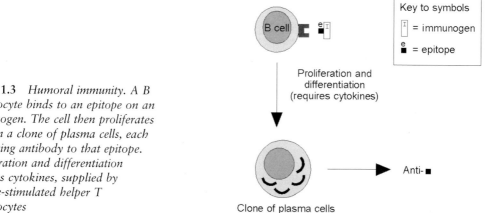

Figure 1.3 *Humoral immunity. A B lymphocyte binds to an epitope on an immunogen. The cell then proliferates to form a clone of plasma cells, each producing antibody to that epitope. Proliferation and differentiation requires cytokines, supplied by epitope-stimulated helper T lymphocytes*

Polyclonal response

A complex immunogen such as a bacterium or a red blood cell has hundreds of proteins and glycoproteins each of which has a number of epitopes. Each epitope will stimulate B cells that have receptors for it and thus a large number of clones of plasma cells will be produced. These plasma cells secrete antibodies of different specificities because they are responding to many different epitopes. Each antibody will bind to the bacterium or the red blood cell but to different epitopes. For this reason, the normal immune response is said to be **polyclonal**.

Activation of T lymphocytes

Unlike B lymphocytes, T lymphocytes do not respond to an antigen in its native state. Instead, they recognize antigen after it has been 'processed' by cells and combined with proteins specified by a region of the genome known as the **major histocompatibility complex (MHC)**. This complex, which is found on chromosome 6 in man, is discussed in Chapter 11. Genes within this region code for two classes of integral membrane proteins, known as Class I and Class II proteins. Class I proteins are found on all the nucleated cells in the body, whereas Class II proteins are restricted to a few cell types. Both Class I and II MHC proteins are initially produced in the cytoplasm where they can bind peptides (either self or 'foreign') and are moved to the membrane. Here they display the peptide to the relevant cells of the immune system.

Each MHC molecule forms a three-dimensional structure in which the bulk of the protein forms a support for a 'peptide-binding groove' into which peptides obtained from proteins can become bound.

Stimulation of T_C cells

The CD8 positive cells that have not yet encountered an immunogen are known as the cytotoxic precursors (T_C) because they give rise, when appropriately stimulated, to the cytotoxic T lymphocytes (CTL). These cells have the capacity to kill cells infected with a virus for which they are specific. Of course, a T_C does not have access to the interior of a virus-infected cell and the mechanism whereby the T_C recognizes that a cell is infected is intriguing. All nucleated cells in the body are able to display portions of the proteins being produced inside them, on their membrane. A healthy cell produces many different proteins in its cytoplasm. Within the cytoplasm, small peptides derived from these proteins become bound to the peptide-binding groove of MHC Class I proteins and from here they are transferred to the membrane. It is only in this form that the T_C can recognize the epitope (that part of the antigen) to which it is specific (see Figure 1.4).

Monoclonal antibodies are the products of a single clone of plasma cells which are producing homogeneous antibodies. They are produced by culturing cells that are actually hybrids of plasma cells, isolated from the spleens of immunized mice, which have been fused to tumour cells to 'immortalize' them. The hybrids grow indefinitely in culture and continue to produce the same antibody. The antibody can be isolated from the supernatants of the cultured cells. Monoclonal antibodies are invaluable in transfusion science because they represent antibodies of a single specificity and a 'reagent' that remains consistent in its qualities. They can be used, for example, in blood grouping, Rhesus D typing and in tissue typing.

It is important to be aware of the difference between polyclonal and monoclonal antibodies and to appreciate that each has advantages and disadvantages.

Figure 1.4   *Cell-mediated immunity. The T-cell receptor on a CD8+ T lymphocyte binds to viral peptide bound to MHC Class I molecules within the cytoplasm and presented on the surface of a virus-infected cell. Binding of the T cell to the peptide is followed by proliferation and differentiation into a clone of cytotoxic T lymphocytes (CTL) capable of killing virus-infected cells directly and indirectly*

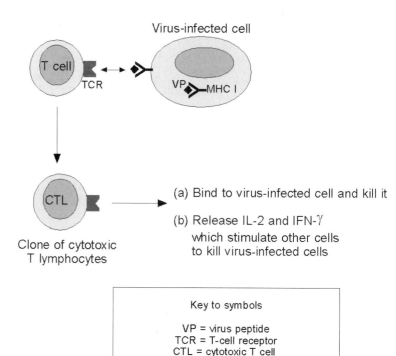

Once the T_C has bound to its epitope in the appropriate manner, it is stimulated to divide many times and develops into a clone of CTL. These cells are similar in appearance to T_C, but have a granular cytoplasm. The granules contain proteins such as **granzymes** and **perforins**, which bring about the destruction of virus-infected cells to which the CTL binds via its specific receptor. Perforins are thought to produce minute 'holes' in the membrane, while granzymes may induce self-destruction by stimulating apoptosis or programmed cell death.

Stimulation of helper T cells

The role of helper T lymphocytes in all aspects of the immune response cannot be overestimated. When stimulated appropriately by an immunogen they secrete cytokines which regulate all aspects of the immune response. Each T_H has epitope-specific receptors that are unable to recognize native antigen. T_H will only recognize an epitope when the antigen is bound in the peptide-binding groove of an MHC Class II molecule in the membrane of a specialized **antigen-presenting cell (APC)**. Very few cell types display Class II MHC molecules. Those that do include monocytes, macrophages, specialized dendritic cells in the blood, interdigitating cells in the lymphoid tissues, and Langerhan's cells in the skin. APC process foreign antigen or 'exogenous' antigen. This means that they take

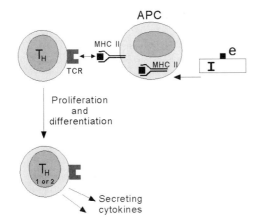

Figure 1.5 *Helper T lymphocytes. An immunogen (I) is taken up into an antigen-presenting cell and processed within the APC. Peptides from the immunogen are bound to MHC Class II molecules and presented at the surface of the APC. Binding of the helper T cell to the foreign peptide is followed by proliferation and differentiation into active helper cells which secrete cytokines*

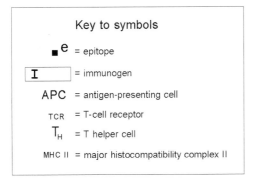

up the immunogen into membrane-bound endosomes. In these endosomes the immunogen is processed by enzymes. Proteins are unfolded and hydrolysed into peptides which then become bound to MHC II molecules (Figure 1.5). The endosome is then transported along microtubules to the cell periphery where the complex becomes inserted into the cell membrane. The helper T lymphocyte only responds to antigen presented in this form.

In addition, the APC also releases IL-1, which seems to be required to stimulate the T_H. When all these conditions are correct, the T_H releases cytokines such as IL-2 which positively stimulates the T_H to divide and to release a whole array of cytokines. Some cytokines are required for the development of humoral immunity and cytotoxic T lymphocytes, while others stimulate non-specific cells such as the macrophages (e.g. IFN-γ) and large granular lymphocytes (e.g. IL-2). Some cytokines (e.g. IL-3) are haemopoeitic factors.

It is thought that there are at least two types of T_H cell according to the cytokines that they secrete (see Table 1.5). The cytokine profiles produced by T_H1 and T_H2 cells promote the production of cell-mediated and humoral immunity, respectively.

Table 1.5   *Cytokine profiles of T_H1 and T_H2 subsets**

	T_H1	T_H2
IL-2	+ + +	−
IFN-γ	+ + +	−
TNF-β	+ + +	−
IL-3	+ + +	+ + +
GM-CSF†	+ +	+ +
IL-4	−	+ + +
IL-5	−	+ + +
IL-6	−	+ +
IL-10	− −	+ + +

* Please note that this is not a complete list of the cytokines produced by T_H cells. In addition, it is thought that T_H1 and T_H2 cells are derived from cells, known as the T_H0 cells, which have a less restricted pattern of cytokine production.

† Granulocyte-macrophage colony stimulating factor – this is a haemopoietic factor which promotes the production of polymorphonuclear leukocytes and monocytes by the bone marrow stem cells.

Suggested further reading

Benjamini, E., Sunshine, G. and Leskowitz, S. (1996). *Immunology A Short Course*, 3rd edn. New York: Wiley-Liss Inc.

Clancy, J. Jr (1998). *Basic Concepts in Immunology: A Student's Survival Guide*. London: McGraw-Hill Health Professions Division.

Roitt, I. (1997). *Essential Immunology*, 9th edn. Oxford: Blackwell Scientific Press.

Self-assessment questions

1. Why is it incorrect to treat non-specific and specific immune mechanisms as entirely separate entities?
2. List the two major features of specific immunity.
3. Why are interferons regarded as cytokines?
4. Name three 'professional phagocytes' and state where they are found in the body. What is the significance of their location?
5. What is the role of inflammation?
6. When might the acute phase response cause harm?
7. What is the relative importance of humoral immunity and cell-mediated immunity in the defence against infection by micro-organisms?
8. Why is a bacterium more immunogenic than a protein?
9. How do B lymphocytes get their name?

10. Why are all small lymphocytes unique prior to antigen stimulation?
11. Why do drugs that inhibit cell division also suppress the immune response?

Key Concepts and Facts

- The immune system consists of a complex set of cells and macromolecules which interact with each other to provide a defence against micro-organisms.

- Inflammation and the acute phase response are non-specific responses to damage and infection.

- Specific immunity involves specificity for an immunogen and immunological memory.

- Small lymphocytes are responsible for specific immunity. They have receptors for epitopes on immunogens.

- B lymphocytes are responsible for humoral immunity (antibody production).

- T_C lymphocytes develop into cytotoxic cells which kill virus-infected cells specifically.

- T_H lymphocytes are responsible for regulating the immune response. They do this by producing proteins called cytokines.

- Immunological responses may also be produced against foreign cells, such as red blood cells and transplanted tissue.

- In autoimmune diseases such as the autoimmune haemolytic anaemias these defences may also be targeted against the individual's own cells and tissue.

Chapter 2
Antibodies and antigens

Learning objectives

After studying this chapter you should confidently be able to:

Classify antibodies into classes and subclasses (where appropriate).

Discuss the properties and outline the functions of different antibody classes.

Describe in detail the structure of IgG.

Show how the structure of IgG relates to the structures of the other antibody classes.

Discuss the molecular forces that allow binding between an antibody and an antigen.

Discuss the significance of antibody affinity and avidity.

Outline the role of antibodies in causing the elimination of an immunogen.

Towards the end of the nineteenth century, evidence had accumulated that, when an individual is immunized, the body manufactures specific defence proteins called antibodies which appear in the blood. Indeed, by 1894, the French scientist Roux had shown that an antiserum from an immunized horse could cure patients with diphtheria. In 1900 Landsteiner used 'naturally occurring' antibodies to distinguish the human A, B and O blood group antigens on the surface of human red blood cells and during the First World War tetanus antitoxin, produced in horses, was injected into recently wounded soldiers to prevent them from developing tetanus.

Despite this long history, the molecular structure of antibodies remained obscure until the Nobel prize-winning work of Porter and Edelman in the late 1950s. These days a great deal is known about antibody structure and function. Such things as where antibodies are formed in the body and the complex cellular interactions which allow them to be manufactured are no longer a mystery. In the 1970s and the years that followed, even the highly complex genetic mechanisms of antibody production which allow so many different antibodies to be produced using a (comparatively) small amount of DNA were beginning to be unravelled. More recently it has been possible to manufacture monoclonal antibodies produced by immunization of B cells *in vitro* or to engineer genetically 'hybrid' antibodies made from a combination of mouse and human genes, which can be used in treating human cancers. The advance of knowledge in this, as in so many areas of immunology, has been phenomenal. This chapter will examine the biochemical nature of antibodies, and how they work.

What antibodies are

Antibodies are glycoproteins, that is, proteins with a significant amount of carbohydrate attached to them. They are found in all the body fluids including plasma, lymph, and secretions such as tears, mucus, saliva and milk. In the blood they appear mostly in the γ globulin fraction (see Figure 2.1) though they extend into the β and α globulin regions. Antibodies are such a heterogeneous group of molecules that they are now known collectively as **immunoglobulins,** i.e. globulins with an immune function. This name was coined by international agreement in 1964, at the same time as they were classified according to their different properties.

Classes of immunoglobulin

Immunoglobulins are classified into five **classes** or **isotypes.** Individuals have antibodies of all five classes in their blood. Antibody classes were first defined by their antigenicity, which means that antibodies raised against one class of immunoglobulin reacted only with that class and no other. The five classes of antibody are all prefixed with **Ig**, standing for immunoglobulin: IgM, IgG, IgA, IgD and IgE. These antibodies differ with respect to their structure, physicochemical properties, their distribution and amount in the body, and their functions. Some properties of these different classes are shown in Table 2.1.

A few useful definitions are given below.

- **Plasma**: The liquid component of blood. Plasma contains proteins, including the clotting factors. It can be obtained from blood by adding an anticoagulant to the blood to prevent clotting and centrifuging the blood to remove the cellular component.

- **Serum**: The liquid component of the blood after it has been allowed to clot; it therefore does not contain clotting factors.

- **Antiserum**: The serum from an animal which has been immunized against an immunogen. It contains antibodies against the immunogen as well as all the other normal components of serum.

- **Antitoxin**: An antiserum directed against a toxoid (a toxin which has been chemically treated to render it harmless).

- **Passive immunization**: The process of injecting antibodies in order to treat or prevent an infectious disease.

- **Active immunization**: The process of injecting an immunogen in order to stimulate a specific immune. response to that immunogen.

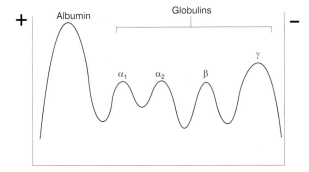

Figure 2.1 *Electrophoresis of plasma. When plasma is subjected to electrophoresis on cellulose acetate at pH 8.6 it separates into several fractions, depending on the charge of the proteins at that pH. Most antibodies are found within the slowest moving fraction, the γ globulin fraction*

Table 2.1   *Properties of different antibody classes*

Class	Mean serum concentration (mg ml^{-1})	Molecular weight (Da)	Carbohydrate (%)
IgM	1.5	900 000	12
IgG	13.5	150 000	2–3
IgA	3.5	160 000–385 000	7–11
IgD	0.03	184 000	9–14
IgE	0.00005	188 000	12

Within some antibody classes, there are also subclasses. Again, these were originally defined by their antigenicity, i.e. while an antiserum raised against the class will react with all the subclasses, there are some antisera which will only react with a particular subclass. These differences in antigenicity reflect basic differences in the amino acid sequences between the subclasses. Humans have four subclasses of IgG and two subclasses of IgA.

Kinetics of the antibody response

Before looking at the structure and function of the different antibody classes, it is necessary to consider the differences between the antibody response in a non-immune and an immune animal. In order to illustrate this, consider an experimental situation in which an animal, such as a rabbit, is immunized with an immunogen such as bovine serum albumin (BSA). The animal is immunized with BSA by injection on day 0 (see Figure 2.2). Samples of blood are taken at daily intervals and the serum tested for the presence of antibodies to the BSA. In an animal that has never been previously immunized with BSA, there is a delay period of approximately 7 days before any anti-BSA can be detected. This delay is known as the **latent period**. After this,

Figure 2.2   *Kinetics of the antibody response. The primary and secondary antibody responses differ in several ways: the length of the latent period (i.e. before antibody is detected), the total amount of antibody, the duration of the response, the predominant class of antibody and the antibody affinity (see text for details)*

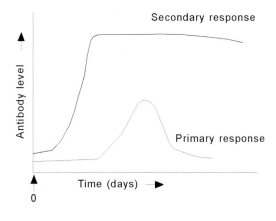

antibody levels reach a peak and then fall to pre-immunization levels by around 21 days. This response, in a non-immune animal, is known as the **primary response**. Most of the antibody produced in a primary response belongs to the IgM class. IgG is only detected towards the end of this response.

When an animal which is immune to BSA (i.e. has already been immunized and gone through a primary response) is re-injected with BSA, a completely different sort of response (**the secondary response**) is seen. There is a shorter latent period, more antibody is produced and the response lasts for much longer (typically weeks or even months). Although IgM is detected at the start of the response, the predominant antibody is IgG. In addition, the antibody produced in a secondary response binds much more strongly to the immunogen, reflecting the production of antibodies with higher **affinity** for the immunogen.

> Knowledge of the kinetics of the antibody response is useful when assessing the immune status of an individual. For example, all pregnant women are tested for antibodies to rubella (German measles). If they have IgM antibodies it probably indicates a recent infection which might have clinical consequences for the baby.
>
> Knowledge of the kinetics of an immune response is also useful when raising antibodies for use, e.g. in clinical studies. IgG is most often required and therefore the antiserum is only taken after a series of immunizations.

Immunoglobulin M

IgM (the M is derived from its original name of β_2 (or γ_1) **macroglobulin**) is always the first antibody to be produced in an immune response and is the predominant antibody of the primary response. Elevated levels of IgM, therefore, usually indicate recent infection. IgM makes up approximately 10% of the immunoglobulins in plasma. The majority of IgM is found in the blood, relatively little being found in lymph and very little in secretions, though traces may be found in milk. IgM is a very effective antibacterial antibody for several reasons, not least its ability to activate complement. The 'naturally occurring' antibodies to the antigens of the ABO blood groups are almost always IgM antibodies. They do not therefore pose any threat to an ABO-incompatible foetus because IgM antibodies do not cross the placenta. However, they are of considerable consequence in the case of ABO-incompatible transfusions (see Chapters 4 and 7).

Immunoglobulin G

IgG is the most abundant antibody in blood and makes up approximately 75% of the immunoglobulins in the plasma. IgG is found in both the vascular and extravascular compartment and is evenly distributed between the two (45 and 55%, respectively). It is the predominant antibody of the secondary response.

IgG is the only antibody which crosses the placenta and it is therefore very important in protecting the developing foetus against infections. Newborn babies have adult levels of IgG in their blood but this is almost entirely of maternal origin. This antibody is catabolized fairly quickly so that, by between 3 and 6 months of age, babies have only low levels of IgG. Thereafter, the levels begin to rise steadily, as the infant is exposed to

> The antibodies of the ABO system are often called 'naturally occurring antibodies' because they are present apparently without immunization with the appropriate red cells. In fact, bacteria also possess antigens of the same type as the A and B antigens and people produce antibodies against these bacterial antigens which they themselves do not have on their red cells (see Chapter 4).

environmental immunogens (and vaccinations) and starts to produce its own IgG. The fact that IgG crosses the placenta has implications for a Rhesus positive foetus developing in a Rhesus negative mother who is already immune to Rhesus positive red blood cells. This can lead to the development of haemolytic disease of the newborn (see Chapter 6).

IgG exists in four **subclasses** (or subisotypes) in man (IgG_{1-4}), the most abundant of which is IgG_1. IgG_3 has a heavier molecular weight but the distribution of the different classes between the vascular and extravascular compartments and the amount of carbohydrate is very similar. These subclasses have complementary roles in the immune response. With the exception of IgG_3, IgG has the longest half-life of the immunoglobulin classes and this persistence makes it suitable for passive immunization, e.g. for treatment of active infection or as a treatment for the prevention of Rhesus isoimmunization (Chapter 6).

Immunoglobulin A

IgA is found in plasma, extravascular fluid and secretions. It exists in different forms depending on where it is located. In humans, most IgA in the serum exists as a 160 000 Da molecule, though a proportion occurs as a dimer of this structure. The vast majority of IgA is found in the secretions and this form is larger. In addition, two subclasses of IgA are found: IgA_1 and IgA_2, the former being the most abundant (3.0 mg ml^{-1} and 0.5 mg ml^{-1} plasma, respectively). The two subclasses have similar distributions and half-lives (approximately 6 days).

While it is not known whether plasma IgA has any significant function, secretory IgA is known to be extremely important in protecting the body from local infections, particularly of mucosal membranes. Far more IgA is made at these sites in total even than the IgG which is secreted into the lymph. Organisms which routinely enter the body via the gut, for example, may be prevented from doing so by the presence of plasma cells in the gut actively secreting IgA. It is therefore important to immunize against these pathogens by local immunization, e.g. oral vaccines against poliomyelitis. IgA is known to be more efficient in the presence of the antibacterial enzyme lysozyme, though the mechanism of this interaction is uncertain.

Immunoglobulin E

IgE is found in low concentrations in serum and has the shortest half-life, a mere 2 days. The low concentrations of free IgE can partly be explained by the fact that IgE has the ability to bind to a receptor on the surface of basophils in the blood and mast cells in the tissues. This receptor is of high affinity so will bind IgE even when the latter is present in such low concentrations. The binding of IgE to these receptors indicates its role in stimulating inflammation (see below) and reflects its importance in helping to eliminate multicellular parasites such as nematodes (roundworms) and helminths from the body. In addition, when produced in response to a 'harmless' immunogen, such as grass pollen, in genetically susceptible individuals, IgE can cause the symptoms of allergies, including hay fever, allergic asthma and food allergies.

Immunoglobulin D

IgD is not considered to have any role as a soluble antibody. This antibody is found in relatively low amounts in plasma where it probably represents IgD receptors which have been shed from the surface of B lymphocytes. All antibody classes can be found as receptors on B lymphocytes and sometimes a cell will display more than one class of receptor. IgD, for example, is frequently found together with IgM.

Structure of IgG

IgG was the first class of antibody to have its structure determined. The work of the British scientist Rodney Porter and the American Gerald Edelman was paramount in this investigation, for which they shared the Nobel prize in 1972. Porter studied the fragments produced when the proteolytic enzymes pepsin and papain were incubated with purified rabbit IgG for limited amounts of time. Edelman studied the effects of mercaptoethanol, which reduces disulphide bonds, on the antibody. When a protein consists of several polypeptide chains held together by disulphide links, mercaptoethanol will reduce these links and cause the chains to fall apart.

The results of their investigations led to the proposal of the structure of IgG that is still held today, which is as follows. A single molecule of IgG consists of four polypeptide chains held together by disulphide links (see Figure 2.3). Two of these chains have a molecular weight of 25 000 Da and are called the light (L) chains. The two light chains in an individual antibody molecule are identical to each other. The other two chains have a molecular weight of 50 000 and are known as the heavy (H) chains. These are also identical to each other. The heavy chains of all IgG molecules have certain similarities in terms of amino acid sequences and are known as γ chains. These are different from the heavy chains of the other classes of antibody. In fact, the classification of antibodies is based on similarities in heavy chain structure within a particular class (see Table 2.2). It is for this reason that antisera raised against IgG heavy chains will not react with IgM heavy chains and vice versa.

When Porter incubated IgG with papain for a limited time, and separated the fragments by ion exchange chromatography, he found that some fragments could still bind a single molecule of antigen. These he called **Fab (Fragment antigen binding)**. The other fragments did not bind antigen but could be crystallized out and he called these **Fc (Fragment crystallizable)**. There were twice as many Fab fragments as Fc. When he digested IgG with pepsin, he obtained a single large fragment which could bind two molecules of hapten and which he called the Fab$'_2$ fragment.

When Edelman treated IgG with mercaptoethanol and separated the chains by gel filtration he obtained two sorts of chains, one half the size of the other. Their molecular weights (see text) indicated that each IgG had two of the 'heavy' chains and two of the 'light' chains.

Figure 2.3 *Structure of an IgG molecule. The molecule consists of heavy (H) and light (L) chains as shown, held together by disulphide links to form two Fab and one Fc site. V and C refer to variable and constant regions, as described in the text. Each variable region consists of a single domain (V_H, V_L) while the constant region has 3 domains (C_H1, C_H2 and C_H3) (see text for details)*

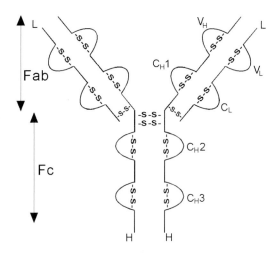

Table 2.2   *The immunoglobulin heavy chains*

Antibody class	Type of heavy chain
IgG	γ
IgM	μ
IgA	α
IgE	ε
IgD	δ

> Have a look at Figure 2.3. Try to predict what will happen if the molecule is broken to the left or the right of the disulphide link between the heavy chains. Now predict where papain and pepsin digest the molecule.

The heavy and light chains are joined together in such a way as to produce a symmetrical molecule with two identical regions known as Fab (Fragment antigen binding) regions and a single Fc (Fragment crystallizable) region. Each Fab region is composed of the light chain and part of the heavy chain. Because an individual IgG molecule has two binding sites it is said to be divalent.

Light chains

By definition, all IgG molecules have γ heavy chains. The situation is different with light chains: only two different forms of light chains exist and these have been designated kappa (κ) light chains and lambda (λ) light chains. They differ in amino acid sequence (all κ chains having certain similarities to other κ light chains and similarly for λ light chains). These light chains may be associated with any of the heavy chain types with the proviso that both the light chains in an individual antibody molecule are always of the same type. Thus an antibody belongs to the IgG class whether it contains two κ chains and two γ chains or two λ chains and two γ chains.

Domain-type structure

In addition to the intrachain disulphide bonds which join the chains together, there are also intrachain disulphide bonds formed between cysteine residues some distance apart in the chain. Bonding between cysteine residues which are separated by approximately 60 amino acids has the effect of forming a loop in the chain. There are four such loops in the γ chain and two in each of the light chains. Each loop occurs within a region known as a **domain** which contains 100–110 amino acids and a single disulphide loop. All immunoglobulins, as well as several other molecules in the immune system, have a similar domain-type structure. Within the domain there is a similar pattern of folding of the polypeptide chain.

Molecules that have this 'domain' structure are thought to be evolutionarily related, having possibly evolved from the same primitive ancestral gene. The molecules are often referred to as the **immunoglobulin superfamily**. They include the T-cell receptor, the CD4 and CD8 molecules on T lymphocytes and the MHC Class I and II molecules which are so important in antigen presentation (see Chapter 1).

Role of the Fab and Fc fragments

The roles of the Fab and Fc regions of an antibody molecule reflect the two main functions of that antibody.

These are:

- To bind to the epitope.
- To stimulate the elimination of the immunogen.

It is the Fab region which binds to the epitope while the Fc region is responsible for mediating the other effector role(s) of the antibody such as activating complement and binding to phagocytic cells. All antibodies are specific for an individual epitope and, for this reason, all antibodies produced by different clones of plasma cells against different epitopes must have different structures. On the other hand, there are relatively few ways in which antibodies can stimulate the elimination of an immunogen and so, in this respect, all antibodies of the same class must be similar in structure. The paradox that all antibodies are different but all antibodies are the same, was neatly confirmed in experiments in which the heavy chains and light chains of many different IgG molecules were analysed for their primary structure, that is, the sequence of amino acids which makes up the polypeptide structures. Analysis of a number of different γ chains revealed that the sequence of amino acids in one section of the heavy chain was very similar in all the chains studied. This sequence constitutes 75% of the γ chain at the C-terminal end of the molecule (approximately 330 amino acids) and is known as the **constant or C region**. It is made up of three domains as shown in Figure 2.3. However, the remaining 25% of the chain, starting at the N-terminal end and comprising a single domain, had an amino acid sequence which differed in all the γ chains studied. This domain is known as the **variable or V region**.

A similar result was found when a number of different κ chains (or λ chains for that matter) was sequenced. In this case, the constant region and variable regions occupy approximately half the light chain at the C-terminal and N-terminal end. Thus, the variability occurs at the Fab end of the molecule. In fact, the antigen-binding site is made up of the variable region of a light chain and a heavy chain. The sequence in each variable region is unique for each antibody that is the product of a different plasma cell. It is this unique sequence which determines the specificity of the antibody. The least variable part of the antibody corresponds to the Fc region, which mediates the other biological functions of the antibody.

Hypervariable regions

When the sequences of a number of variable regions on κ, λ or γ chains were analysed in more depth, it was discovered that there were different degrees of variability even within the variable regions. For example, the sequences of a number of variable regions of γ chains revealed that some parts of these regions were even more variable than the rest. There were three such hypervariable regions for every V region studied (whether light or heavy) and these are very important structures for determining the specificity of the antibody. They are nowadays referred to as the **complementarity determining regions** (CDR) and the six CDRs in each Fab region (three from the heavy and three from the light chain) give the binding site a unique 'shape' into which only the epitope will fit well. The 'less variable' regions between and around the CDRs are called the **'framework'** regions, and they support the CDRs which form the shape of the binding site.

Binding of antibody to the epitope

At this point, a little revision might be useful. Remember that an epitope is a small region of an immunogen to which an antibody binds. It may be a short sequence of a protein (about five to seven amino acids in size), or an oligosaccharide forming part of a glycoprotein (the antigens of the ABO system for example; see Chapter 5) or it may be a hapten, a molecule which has been deliberately attached to a protein in order to stimulate antibody production. In essence, the epitope is relatively small compared with the whole antibody molecule but not necessarily when compared to the antibody-binding site. Remember, too, that the term antigen is given to a molecule which combines with an antibody, and is often used when discussing reactions occurring *in vitro*. Both terms will be used in this chapter.

The antibody binding site

The interaction between an antibody and an epitope has been likened to a 'lock and key' mechanism, where the epitope is the 'key' and the binding site is the 'lock'. Essentially, the prime consideration as to whether an antibody will bind an epitope is

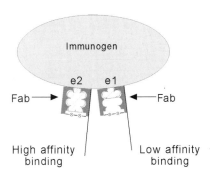

Figure 2.4 *Antigen/antibody binding. When the Fab site is complementary in shape to the epitope, high affinity binding can occur. Alternatively, an epitope may fit less well into the binding site, to give low affinity binding*

Table 2.3 *Forces holding the antibody/antigen together*

Force	Origin
Hydrophobic interactions	Between molecules that come together because they mutually expel water
Hydrogen bonds	Where hydrogen is shared between electronegative atoms such as nitrogen and oxygen
Electrostatic interaction	Between oppositely charged groups
Van der Waal's forces	Interactions between electron clouds around molecules

the complementarity between the shape of the binding site and the shape of the epitope (see Figure 2.4). When they are complementary, the epitope will fit well into the binding site, allowing amino acid residues in the antibody to fit closely to residues making up the epitope, and allowing secondary interactions to take place which stabilize the binding. These other forces are described in Table 2.3. Note that there are no covalent interactions between the antibody and the epitope. The reaction is reversible and is governed by the law of mass action. However, if there is good fit between the antibody and the epitope, there will be high affinity binding and separating the two molecules will be difficult to achieve.

Antibody affinity

The binding of an antibody-binding site to the epitope is a chemical reaction and can be defined by certain characteristics. One of the most useful is the term **affinity**. This is a precise chemical description which is a measure of the strength of binding of a single antibody-binding site to a univalent antigen (i.e. one with only one epitope). The affinity of an antibody is an important property and it governs, for example, whether or not this antibody will be useful *in vitro* for the detection of blood group antigens or, *in vivo*, the pathological consequences of a particular, unwanted antibody, such as an antibody to red blood cells in haemolytic anaemia.

Consider the following reaction: antibody + antigen $\rightleftharpoons$ immune complex, or:

$$Ab + Ag \rightleftharpoons AbAg$$

According to the law of mass action, the rate of the forward reaction is proportional to the concentration of the reactants:

$$r_1 \propto [Ab] \times [Ag]$$

$$r_1 = k_1[Ab] \times [Ag] \text{ where } k_1 \text{ is the rate}$$
constant for the forward reaction

Conversely, the rate of the backward reaction (r_2) is proportional to the concentration of the product:

$$r_2 = k_2 [AbAg]$$

At equilibrium the rates of the forward and backward reactions are balanced and $r_1 = r_2$; and therefore:

$$k_1 [Ab] \times [Ag] = k_2 [AbAg]$$

and

$$k_1/k_2 = [AbAg]/[Ag] \times [Ag]$$

The figure k_1/k_2 is the **association constant**, K, or **affinity** and its units are $l\,mol^{-1}$ when the concentrations of the reactants are given in $mol\,l^{-1}$. An antibody with an association constant of $10^5\,l\,mol^{-1}$ does not bind as strongly as an antibody with an affinity of $10^7\,l\,mol^{-1}$.

Sometimes the term affinity is expressed as the reciprocal of K. This has units of concentration and is in many ways more easy to understand. For example, a figure for $1/K$ of 10^{-8} M would indicate a concentration of the antigen required in order to ensure that half the antibody binding sites were occupied. In this case the lower the concentration of antigen required to achieve 50% binding, the higher the affinity.

The affinity, as defined above, refers to the binding of a homogeneous antibody to a single epitope or a univalent antigen, such as a hapten. Apart from monoclonal antibodies, antibodies produced in animals are very heterogeneous, because they are the product of a polyclonal response. The affinity that is actually measured in such a preparation is the average of the affinities of all the antibodies in that preparation and K is the **average association constant**.

Avidity

Most immunogens have many different epitopes. An antiserum prepared against such an immunogen will contain antibodies against many epitopes and there will be a range of antibodies of different affinities against all these different epitopes. Measuring the strength of binding of an antiserum against a multivalent antigen is therefore less precise than measuring the reaction between the binding of a single antibody and a single epitope. The term **avidity** is used to denote the strength of binding between antibodies and multivalent antigens or immunogens. In addition, the number of Fab sites on the antibody is also important in determining the strength of binding. For example, when comparing IgG with IgM, even if individual binding sites on these antibodies have the same affinity for an epitopes, IgM will bind to an immunogen containing repeated epitopes with higher avidity simply because it has 10 binding sites, while IgG has only two.

Structure of IgM

As was previously mentioned, the heavy chains of IgM are larger than those of IgG and this is because they have an extra domain in the constant region, i.e. they have one variable and four constant domains. However, the increase in the size of the heavy chains alone cannot account for the molecular weight of 900 000. The difference between these immunoglobulins is based on the fact that IgM is polymeric, where the monomeric unit is the basic four-chain structure as already discussed with reference to IgG. IgM is actually a pentamer, containing five of these four-chain units (see Figure 2.5). The five units are joined together through disulphide links between the Fc regions and through an additional protein, the J-chain (molecular weight 15 000 Da), which links two of the four-chain structures. The J-chain is produced within the plasma cell and assembled along with the heavy and light chains.

Theoretically, a pentameric IgM having 10 Fab sites should be able to bind 10 molecules of the epitope. In practice, the number bound is nearer to five, and this seems to be due to constraints of size: there is not enough room to 'fit' 10 epitopes around the molecule.

Immunoglobulins A, E and D

The majority of plasma IgA in humans is present in a monomeric form. However, it can also exist as a dimer, which is held together through disulphide bonds and a J-chain (see Figure 2.5). Secretory IgA also occurs as a dimer held together by a J-chain, but with an additional protein, **the secretory component**, wrapped around the joined Fc regions of the dimer. This secretory component (molecular weight 70 000 Da) is produced by epithelial cells through which IgA passes as it is secreted. Secretory component probably serves to protect the antibody from the action of proteolytic enzymes in hostile environments such as the gut. It is also possible that this component actually facilitates secretion.

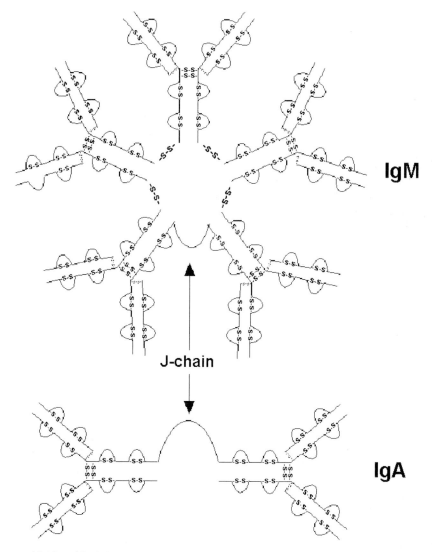

Figure 2.5 *Structure of IgM and IgA. IgM is a pentamer made up of five four-chain 'units' linked by a J-chain and by disulphide bonds. IgA may take the form of a dimer linked by a J-chain*

IgE has a monomeric form. Its large molecular weight (188 000 Da) reflects the larger heavy chains which, like the μ chains of IgM, have an additional constant region domain. IgE molecules are also fairly heavily glycosylated, though the precise role of the carbohydrate is not certain.

IgD is found in very low concentrations in the plasma, though it is more abundant as a membrane-associated B-cell receptor. Its relatively large molecular weight is not due to extra domains but to an extended hinge region. This antibody has a short half-life owing to an extreme susceptibility to enzymic proteolysis.

Table 2.4 *Effector activities of antibodies*

Activity	Antibodies involved
Bring about physical changes to the immunogen, e.g. agglutination of cells, precipitation of proteins	IgM, IgG, IgA
Trigger lysis of cellular immunogens	IgM, IgG
Trigger inflammation	IgM, IgG, IgE
Increase the efficiency of uptake and destruction by phagocytic cells	IgM, IgG, IgA

Effector role of the antibody

The secondary role of the antibody is stimulated following binding to the immunogen. Various activities may be stimulated following binding and these are summarized in Table 2.4. The importance of each of these activities depends to a certain extent on the location of the antigen/antibody reaction, on the nature of the immunogen, and on the class of antibody involved.

Physical changes

An antibody binding to a soluble immunogen, such as a toxin, can precipitate the protein out of solution. This happens if antibody and antigen are present in the proportions needed to produced a large lattice-like complex of antibodies and antigens. Precipitation depends upon the antigen being multivalent (having several epitopes) and having sufficient antibody to produce the 'optimal proportions' required. *In vivo* this may serve the purpose of making the complex more easily phagocytosed. Only those antibodies normally present in sufficient concentration may be regarded as precipitating, i.e. IgM, IgG and IgA (see Figure 2.6).

When an antibody is directed against a cell rather than a soluble protein, the combination may cause the cells to clump together or **agglutinate**. IgM is the most efficient agglutinating antibody. Indeed IgG is unable to agglutinate red cells directly owing to the negative surface charge of these cells and this will be discussed in some detail in Chapter 8.

Lysis

Antibodies may cause lysis of cellular immunogens in two different ways.

- By activating complement: In effect, antibodies binding to the membranes of cells activate a series of reactions that result in lysis. IgM is the most efficient lytic antibody, though IgG can also activate complement. In blood transfusion reactions, much of the

The physical changes brought about when an antibody combines with an antigen can be used in tests to detect either antigen or antibody. For example, precipitation tests are used to quantify plasma proteins. Examples of these tests are nephelometry, radial immunodiffusion and rocket electrophoresis. IgG and IgM can effectively agglutinate bacteria and, even today, a number of laboratory tests to determine immune status to a micro-organism are based on agglutination. Antibodies are very discriminatory and have allowed the classification of bacteria into species, groups, subgroups and strains. Agglutination tests are the most common tests used in transfusion science.

Figure 2.6 *Secondary role of the antibody. An antibody may precipitate soluble proteins (a) or agglutinate cells (b) by forming multiple crosslinks between the molecules of antigen and antibody. IgG may lyse cells (c) by binding via the Fc region to large granular lymphocytes (LGL), stimulating the latter to release perforins*

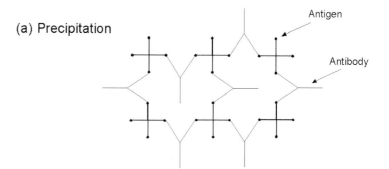

(a) Precipitation

Antigen

Antibody

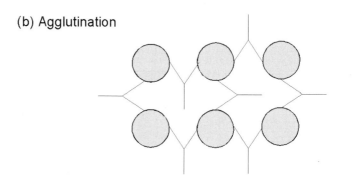

(b) Agglutination

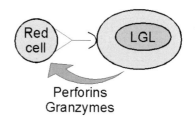

(c) ADCC

Red cell

LGL

Perforins
Granzymes

pathology involves the activation of complement. This topic is discussed in some detail in Chapter 3.

- By triggering the activity of large granular lymphocytes (LGL): LGL have membrane-bound receptors for the Fc region of IgG (FcγR). Thus, when an IgG molecule binds to a cell via its Fab region, the Fc region will bind to the LGL. When this happens, the LGL is triggered to release proteins in its granular cytoplasm which destroy the membrane of the target cell (see Figure 2.6). This type of killing is known as **antibody-dependent cellular cytotoxicity (ADCC)** and is only mediated by IgG. The process is very efficient in terms of the amount of antibody required, which is, in theory, a single antibody molecule per target cell. ADCC can also be carried out by monocytes and has been used to test for the clinical significance of anti-Rh antibodies.

Stimulation of inflammation

The binding of antibodies to an antigen may stimulate inflammation in two different ways.

- Through the activation of complement: When complement is activated by IgG or IgM bound to an antigen, a number of pharmacologically active proteins are produced. Some of these components have **anaphylatoxin** activity. This means that they bind to mast cells in the tissues and basophils in the blood and stimulate them to degranulate. The histamine released from these cells triggers inflammation. The inflammatory process serves both to allow plasma (containing complement and antibodies) to enter an inflammatory site and may also result in the exudation of neutrophils into the inflamed area, thus promoting phagocytosis.
- IgE-induced inflammation: Mast cells and basophils have high affinity receptors for the Fc region of IgE (FcεR). Much of the IgE that is produced in the body becomes bound to these receptors. Degranulation of mast cells and basophils is triggered when an antigen crosslinks two specific IgE molecules on the surface of these cells. The histamine released triggers inflammation. Other pharmacologically active agents are also released which, together with histamine, cause a variety of effects including smooth muscle contraction, increased mucus secretion and the accumulation of eosinophils at the site of release.

Stimulation of phagocytosis

The binding of antibodies to an antigen may stimulate phagocytosis in several ways.

- Through the antibody receptor on phagocytic cells: Receptors for the Fc region of IgG are widely distributed on phagocytic cells. Three different types of FcγR are now recognized. In addition, phagocytic cells may also have receptors for the Fc regions of other antibodies such as IgA. When IgG has bound to an antigen, the complex is preferentially bound to the Fc receptor on the phagocytic cell. This has the effect of not just bringing the antigen and the phagocyte together but also amplifying many of the activities of the phagocyte including uptake of antigen, the respiratory burst and the production of hypochlorite.
- By activating complement: This can occur in several ways. For example, some activated complement proteins are chemotactic factors for neutrophils. Phagocytic cells also have receptors for a variety of complement proteins, including products of activation of C3. Thus, complement can also opsonize antigens and stimulate uptake by phagocytes. Red blood cells also have C3 receptors, enabling them to pick up immune complexes and transport them to the spleen and liver, where the complexes are

IgE-induced inflammation is involved in the elimination of multicellular parasites since these cannot be lysed and are too big to be engulfed by phagocytes. Unfortunately, IgE may sometimes be produced in response to inappropriate antigens such as pollen and the faeces of house-dust mites. This leads to the development of hay fever and allergic asthma. Sufferers of these syndromes will recognize the effects of histamine.

stripped from their surfaces and phagocytosed by macrophages. This is an important mechanism for removal of complexes owing to the large numbers of red cells in the blood.

Suggested further reading

Abbas, A.K., Lichtman, A.H. and Pober, J.S. (1997). Antibodies and antigens. In *Cellular and Molecular Immunology*. Philadelphia: W.B. Saunders Company.

Burton, D.R. (1990). Antibody: the flexible adapter molecule. *Trends in Biochemical Science*, **15**, 64–69.

French, M.A.H. (1986). *Immunoglobulins in Health and Disease*. Lancaster: MTP.

Steward, M. and Male, D. (1998). Immunological techniques. In *Immunology*, 5th edn (eds Roitt, Brostoff and Male). London: Mosby.

Self-assessment questions

1. Which of the immunoglobulins is:
   (a) The most abundant in blood?
   (b) Always produced first in an immune response?
   (c) Involved in the elimination of parasites?
   (d) The most abundant in secretions?
2. What is the basis for classifying the immunoglobulins?
3. Why is IgG used for passive immunization?
4. State two ways in which the structure of IgM differs from that of IgG.
5. Distinguish between the constant and variable regions of heavy chains.
6. Name two roles of the Fc region of IgG.
7. List three forces involved in the binding of an antibody to an antigen.
8. Distinguish between the terms affinity and avidity.
9. Name two ways in which IgG can promote phagocytosis.

Key Concepts and Facts

- Antibodies are immunoglobulins found in the blood, extra-vascular fluid and secretions. They are produced by stimulated B lymphocytes.

- Antibodies have a dual role: they bind to an immunogen and stimulate its elimination.

- The structure of antibodies is such that it provides both the specificity of binding and the 'common' role of elimination within the same structure.

- There are five classes of antibody which differ in structure, location and immunological role.

- Antibodies against red cells usually belong to the IgG or IgM classes.

- By binding to red cells antibodies trigger their lysis and uptake by phagocytic cells as well as stimulating inflammatory reactions. These manifestations are evident in transfusion reactions and immune haemolytic anaemias.

Chapter 3
Complement

Learning objectives

After studying this chapter you should confidently be able to:

State what complement is and where it is found.

Recognize the difference between classical and alternative pathway activation.

Discuss the major pathways for classical and alternative activation.

Discuss the lytic sequence.

Discuss the role of complement in stimulating inflammation and phagocytosis.

Briefly discuss how complement is measured.

Recognize the uses of complement as a reagent in the transfusion laboratory.

Towards the end of the nineteenth century, several scientists recorded the presence of a heat-labile substance in fresh serum which was able to **complement** the activity of antibodies. For example, Buchner in 1893 showed that serum which was able to kill certain bacteria lost this ability after it had been heated to 56°C. In 1895 Bordet, to whom the discovery of complement is often attributed, showed that the ability of an antiserum to kill the bacteria which cause cholera depended on the presence of a heat-labile substance as well as the antibodies. This substance, first called **alexine**, is now better known as **complement**. By the beginning of the twentieth century it became clear that the same substance was also required for the antibody-mediated lysis of red blood cells. Today, complement is important to the transfusion scientist for several reasons. It is a substance that is involved in the pathology of the immune and drug-induced haemolytic anaemias, and in blood transfusion reactions. In addition, complement is also useful as a biological reagent in demonstrating the presence of potentially lytic antibodies and detecting clinically significant complement-binding blood group antibodies. This chapter will discuss the activation of complement, its role in immune elimination, and its involvement in haemolytic disorders.

Complement is not a single entity

The name complement refers to a set of at least 16 different proteins found in the blood plasma and lymph which carry out the following roles:

- Lysing (literally splitting open) red cells and other 'target' cells.
- Stimulating inflammation.
- Attracting phagocytic cells into an infected area.
- Stimulating phagocytosis.
- Clearing of immune (antigen/antibody) complexes.

Thus, complement is important in killing target cells, such as bacteria, and for aiding the immune system in the disposal of the remains using the phagocytic cells. It also stimulates the lysis and phagocytic destruction of antibody-coated red cells in transfusion reactions, haemolytic disease etc.

Owing to the lytic and inflammatory potential of complement proteins, these proteins are usually present in an inactive form, often as proenzymes, requiring conversion to an active enzyme. In other words, complement has to be **activated** to fulfil its role. In addition to the proteins that are involved in these activities, there are a number of proteins that regulate the actions of complement. For example, there are proteins which help to prevent the lysis of the body's own cells.

Activation pathways

There are two major pathways for the activation of complement. These are known as the **classical pathway** and the **alternative pathway**. Both these activation pathways feed into a common pathway which results in the lysis of the target cell. They also both result in the production of proteins which induce phagocytosis and inflammation (see Figure 3.1). The alternative pathway is a first line of defence against micro-organisms, because it is activated by the cell wall components of these cells, in the absence of antibody (see Table 3.1). This pathway is dependent on the presence of magnesium ions. The classical pathway is initiated when antibody binds to an antigen and may therefore take several days to be effective, if specific antibody is not already present. The classical pathway is dependent on the presence of both magnesium and calcium ions.

The proteins involved in the two activation pathways and in the lytic sequence are shown in Table 3.2. Unfortunately, the numbering system does not follow the chronological sequence of

The sequences that involve activation of proenzymes are very important to the activity of complement. In such cases, several molecules of a proenzyme are cleaved by a previous component in the sequence to yield two fragments, 'a' and 'b', one of which (usually 'b') becomes a new enzyme. There are now several molecules of 'b' each of which is able to cleave many molecules of the next proenzyme to yield even more molecules of the next enzyme. Thus there is **amplification** in the system. When a complement protein is cleaved into two fragments, 'a' and 'b', on most occasions the 'b' fragment is the largest. The exception to this rule is C2, which is cleaved into a larger C2a and a smaller C2b.

Figure 3.1 *Complement may be activated by two different pathways, both of which can converge, resulting in lysis of a foreign cell and the release of inflammatory mediators*

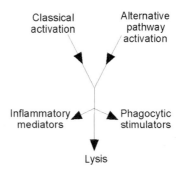

Table 3.1 *Activators of complement*

Classical pathway	*Alternative pathway*
IgG bound to antigen	Lipopolysaccharide (bacterial cell walls)
IgM	Zymosan (yeast cell walls)
C-reactive protein	Heat aggregated IgA
Heat aggregated IgG	Trypanosomes
	Cobra venom factor (CVF)
	Some virus-infected cells
	Inulin*

* Inulin is a polysaccharide obtained from the Jerusalem artichoke! This has very little significance to us *in vivo* but the carbohydrate is often used as an alternative pathway activator *in vitro*.

The names 'classical' and 'alternative' may give the impression that the latter is less important than the former. This is not the case since, in terms of speed, the alternative pathway is activated more rapidly, because it does not rely on the presence of antibody. The classical pathway was, in fact, the first to be discovered. The alternative pathway was recognized much later, though it is probably more primitive in evolutionary terms. In 1954, Louis Pillemer added zymosan from yeast cell walls to fresh serum and showed that this serum could not longer lyse antibody-coated target cells. This implied that the complement had been 'used up' or **fixed** by something other than antibody.

complement activation. It was also discovered, some time after its naming, that C1, the first component of complement, was actually a complex of three different proteins and these were subsequently named **C1q, C1r** and **C1s.** These proteins are present in the molecular ratio of 1:2:2. They are loosely associated with each other and held together through calcium ions. Complement proteins are produced by a number of cells. The hepatocytes in the liver produce most of the C3, C6, C7 and C9 found in the plasma. During an acute phase response (see Chapter 1) their production is greatly increased. Macrophages produce C1q, C1r and C1s, C2, C4 and C5.

The classical pathway: activation to lysis

The first step in the classical pathway occurs when an antibody binds to an antigen. The only antibodies that can activate complement by this pathway are IgM and IgG. In order to examine complement activation from the point of view of a transfusion scientist, the sequence will be discussed as if an antibody was binding to an antigen on the surface of a red cell. However, this could equally well be happening at the membrane of a bacterial

Table 3.2 *Complement proteins*

Protein	Molecular weight (Da)	Classical or alternative activation pathway or lytic sequence
C1q	410 000	Classical
C1r	190 000	Classical
C1s	87 000	Classical
C2	115 000	Classical
C3	180 000	Classical and alternative
C4	210 000	Classical
C5	190 000	Lytic
C6	128 000	Lytic
C7	121 000	Lytic
C8	163 000	Lytic
C9	79 000	Lytic
Factor B	93 000	Alternative
Factor D	24 000	Alternative
Factor H	150 000	Alternative
Factor I	88 000	Alternative
Factor P	220 000	Alternative

cell. Complement is also activated when antibody binds to a soluble immunogen, such as a toxin, though obviously this will not result in lysis.

The complement proteins involved in classical activation are **C1, C2, C4** and **C3** (in that order), and in the lytic cycle **C5, C6, C7, C8** and **C9**. The starting point for activation of the classical pathway occurs when IgG or IgM binds to an antigen on the red cell membrane. Activation of this pathway requires enough antibody to be present on the membrane such that two Fc regions are sufficiently close to bind the same molecule of C1q (see Figure 3.2). IgM is very efficient at activating or **fixing** complement because each molecule has five Fc regions close together. IgG, on the other hand, has only one Fc region per molecule and it has been estimated that approximately 1000 molecules of IgG must bind to a red cell in order to achieve the density required for activation to occur.

C1q is a large protein (Table 3.2). Its three-dimensional structure, seen on electron micrographs, has been likened to a bunch of six tulips which are all fused at the stalks. Each of the 'flowers' is able to bind to a site on the Fc region of the antibody. The site to which the C1q binds is located on the C_H2 domain of IgG and the C_H3 domain of IgM (see Chapter 2). All that is required to activate complement is for two of the 'tulip heads' to become bound to adjacent Fc regions at the red cell membrane. This binding is facilitated by the 'tulip stalks' which contain collagen-like protein sequences and are very flexible.

Not all IgG subclasses bind complement: IgG_3 activates more than IgG_1, with IgG_2 being much less effective and IgG_4 not binding at all. Thus, a blood group antibody which is of the IgG_4 subclass will not be detected by methods that depend on complement binding.

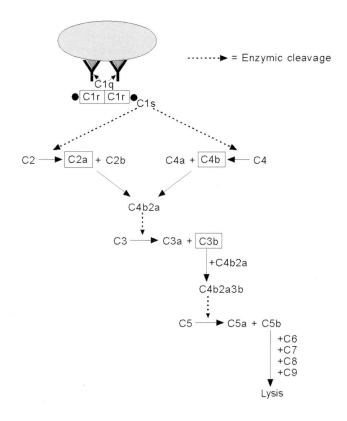

Figure 3.2 *Classical pathway for complement activation. Binding of C1q to two adjacent Fc regions on the surface of a red cell initiates a series of reactions, resulting in lysis of the red cell. These reactions are described in the text*

Prior to activation all complement proteins are dissolved in the plasma, i.e. the fluid phase.

In order to lyse a cell, complement proteins have to be recruited onto the membrane of the target cell. There are several steps in the activation process in which complement proteins are taken out of the fluid phase and recruited to the target cell membrane, the first being when C1q binds to the Fc region of the antibody which is itself bound to the target cell membrane.

The production of a C3 splitting enzyme, or convertase, is pivotal to both the classical and the alternative pathways. However, although both pathways produce such an enzyme, they are not actually the same molecules.

The binding of C1q in this manner results in the activation of the C1r component. C1r acquires enzymatic activity and cleaves a peptide from C1s to expose the active site of this proteolytic enzyme. Thus activated C1s is a proteolytic enzyme able to cleave C4 into two fragments, C4a and C4b. C4b has a hydrophobic binding site which allows it to bind to the red cell membrane. It binds at membrane sites other than those already occupied by antibody. This is only a short-term (transient) binding site. Any C4b which fails to bind to the red cell continues the sequence in the plasma.

C1s also acts on the next complement component, C2, and cleaves it into two fragments, C2a and C2b. The larger fragment, C2a, binds to C4b at the red cell membrane in the presence of magnesium ions to form a new enzyme, **C4b2a**. The smaller fragments, C4a and C2b, remain in the plasma. The new enzyme C4b2a is otherwise known as **classical pathway C3 convertase** because it is capable of cleaving C3 into two fragments, C3a and C3b.

C3b contains most of the structure of C3, with the exception of a 9000 Da fragment (C3a) sliced off one of the two polypeptide chains which make up this protein. C3a has important inflammatory properties which are discussed below. When first produced, C3b, like C4b, has a transient binding site which allows it to bind to

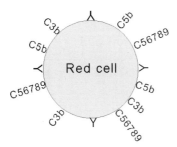

Figure 3.3 *Consequences of complement activation. A red cell coated with antibody becomes coated with a variety of activated complement proteins, each with biological activity. Moreover, there are far more of these molecules on the red cell surface than molecules of the antibody which triggered activation, i.e. amplification has occurred*

the red cell membrane or to the C3 convertase (C4b2a). C3b which fails to bind to the membrane continues the sequence in the plasma.

Whether it is attached to the red cell or not, a molecule of C3b which binds to a molecule of the C3 convertase (C4b2a) produces a new enzyme, **C4b2aC3b**, which is a **C5 convertase**. This enzyme cleaves C5 into two fragments, C5a and C5b. C5a has important inflammatory properties which will be discussed later. C5b also has a transient hydrophobic binding site which allows it to bind to the target cell membrane. At this stage the red cell has numerous proteins attached to the membrane at different sites. These proteins include antibody, C1q, C4b, C4b2a, C3b, C4b2aC3b and C5b (see Figure 3.3). All steps up to this stage are enzymic and much amplification occurs so that there may be thousands of molecules of C5b attached to the membrane. It is at the sites where C5b has bound that the pores in the membrane which will eventually result in haemolysis are produced.

The following stages are not enzymic, but involve the sequential addition, to C5b, of a molecule each of C6, C7 and C8, and several copies of C9. This produces a very large molecular weight (> 1 000 000 Da) complex called the **membrane attack complex (MAC)**. Each MAC is built up at the membrane as a set of hydrophobic proteins lining a cylinder. The cylinder becomes inserted into the membrane of the target cells and a pore is produced. The process of pore formation has not been fully determined, though several theories have been suggested. The pores themselves have a diameter of approximately 10 nm. They allow the passage of ions and small molecules to occur between the cell and its environment such that the normal gradients of these molecules across the cell membrane are lost, and equilibration occurs. However, since large molecules such as proteins are too big to leak out of the cell, a high osmotic pressure is built up within the cell, allowing water to cross the undamaged membrane by osmosis. This influx of water kills the cell.

Lysis of antibody-coated cells is most spectacularly seen with red cells, which literally burst following the activation of the classical pathway. *In vitro* this can be seen as a sudden 'clearing' of a previously cloudy cell suspension, due to the release of haemoglobin from the cells. With other types of mammalian cells the reaction is

The presence of a very short-term binding site helps to ensure that C3b only binds to cells near to where it was produced, i.e. the target cell to which the C1q has become bound. Binding of C3b to 'self' cells would ultimately result in injury to those cells.

When an antibody-coated red blood cell becomes coated with complement proteins following complement activation, there is very much more complement on the red blood cell than the antibody which triggered it in the first place. This is due to amplification. Therefore, in a transfusion laboratory, it is always much easier to detect complement on red blood cells than to detect antibodies. The presence of activated complement proteins on red blood cells is used as an **indicator** of the presence of complement-binding antibodies.

Any C5b which fails to bind to the membrane can continue the sequence in the fluid phase. There is the possibility that complexes of C5b67 can bind to innocent bystander cells and initiate lysis. Such a situation is called **reactive lysis**. Reactive lysis may amplify the effects of any unwanted antibody, such as an antibody to red blood cells.

not so dramatic and the cells die without necessarily bursting immediately. These cells can be shown to be dead by staining them with dyes which are normally excluded from cells with intact, healthy membranes (see details of tissue typing in Chapter 9).

Other biological activities of complement

The lytic activity of complement is not its major defence role *in vivo*, though it is a very useful end-point in *in vitro* assays and, as previously mentioned, plays a strong part in the pathology of transfusion reactions and haemolytic anaemias. Other important roles of complement include opsonization, attracting phagocytes, stimulating inflammation and clearing immune complexes, and these may be more significant with respect to the beneficial role of complement in eliminating micro-organisms from the body.

Opsonization and clearance of immune complexes

Phagocytic cells, including neutrophils, monocytes and macro-phages, have receptors for C3b. Thus, a cell which has become coated with C3b will bind to these receptors, a phenomenon known as **immune adherence**. C3b-coated red cells may also bind to surfaces such as the walls of blood vessels, making them easy targets for phagocytic cells in the blood. There are various forms of complement receptor (CR) which bind C3b and its derivatives (see Table 3.3).

Binding of the complement-coated cell to the phagocyte in this way activates the phagocyte so that it is more efficient at ingesting and destroying cells. Metabolism of the phagocyte is also enhanced.

Table 3.3 *Complement receptors*

Receptor	Complement proteins bound	Distribution
CR1	C3b, C4b, C3bi*	Red cells, eosinophils, neutrophils, monocytes, macrophages, B cells, some T cells, follicular dendritic cells (in lymph nodes)
CR2	C3bi, C3dg*, C3d*	B cells, follicular dendritic cells
CR3	C3bi	Neutrophils, NK cells, monocytes, macrophages, follicular dendritic cells
CR4	C3bi	Neutrophils, monocytes, macrophages, platelets

* These proteins are various forms of inactivated C3b. They are discussed with the alternative pathway in the text.

C3b can also become bound to soluble immune complexes, favouring their binding to, and subsequent uptake by, the phagocytes. Red blood cells also have CR1 receptors in their membranes so that C3b-coated cells bind to circulating red blood cells and are removed by phagocytes in the liver and the spleen. Each red blood cell has far fewer CR1 receptor molecules per cell than a phagocyte, but this does not mean that their role is insignificant since there are approximately 1000 red blood cells for every leukocyte. It has been calculated that, collectively, red blood cells have 90% of the CR1 molecules in the blood and are therefore very important in removing immune complexes from the blood stream.

Attracting phagocytes

The proteins C3a and C5a are chemotactic for neutrophils. This means that neutrophils will be attracted to any area where complement is activated. It is this activity which is thought to play a significant role in the build up of neutrophils at a site of inflammation, particularly when bacteria have entered that site.

The complex C5b67 is also known to be chemotactic for neutrophils.

Stimulation of inflammation

C3a, C5a and, to a lesser extent, C4a have **anaphylatoxin** activity. This means that they bind to blood basophils and tissue mast cells and cause them to degranulate. The histamine released then triggers vasodilatation, allowing more plasma (containing complement, antibodies etc.) to get into the inflamed site. In addition, the dilated blood vessel allows the neutrophils to gain access to the site to which they have been chemotactically attracted. It is also known that C5a binds to macrophages, inducing them to release IL-1 and IL-6, both of which are known to increase the expression of **cell adhesion molecules** (CAMs) on the surface of the endothelial cells which line the blood vessel. These CAMs are necessary for the adherence of neutrophils to the blood vessel and for their migration between the endothelial cells and into the inflamed site. IL-1 and IL-6 also stimulate the bone marrow to release neutrophil reserves during an acute phase response. Thus it can be seen that all the different responses to damage and infection are very much inter-related.

Interaction of complement with other systems

Complement is known to interact with several other systems, including the blood clotting system to promote aggregation of platelets, and the fibrinolytic system resulting in the dissolution of blood clots. The former may contribute to some of the pathology seen in transfusion reactions. The reader who wishes to learn more about the wealth of complement activities is advised to see the suggested reading at the end of this chapter.

Alternative pathway for complement activation

The alternative pathway for complement activation is actually not a pathway at all, but is a **positive feedback loop.** It is an amplification system which increases C3 breakdown, whenever C3b has been produced. An alternative pathway activator can then be seen as anything that increases the activity of this 'loop'. This amplification loop, and its regulation, is shown in Figure 3.4.

Whenever C3b has been produced, perhaps from the classical pathway or perhaps by a very slow natural breakdown of C3 into C3a and C3b, this C3b can enter the amplification loop. The protein, Factor B, which is present in plasma binds to C3b to form a complex, C3bB. The Factor B that forms part of this complex is then cleaved by a plasma enzyme known as Factor D, releasing the smaller fragment, Ba, and leaving Bb as part of the complex, which is known as C3bBb. This complex is the **alternative pathway C3 convertase** and catalyses the cleavage of more C3 into

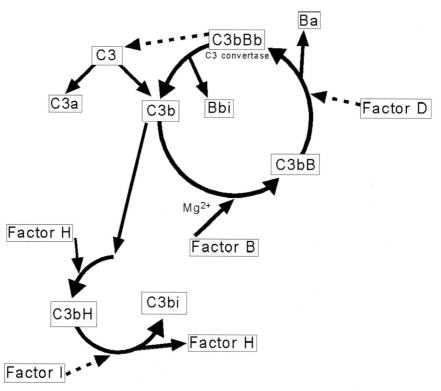

Figure 3.4 *Alternative pathway for complement activation. The alternative pathway involves a positive amplification loop in which C3b positively stimulates the breakdown of more C3. Details of this pathway and its control are described in the text*

C3a and C3b. If this feedback loop were uncontrolled, then the plasma content of C3 would very rapidly be exhausted due to its breakdown, and more and more C3b would appear on cell surfaces. However, there are several control points:

- The enzyme C3bBb is inherently unstable and breaks down to produce C3b and an inactive form of Bb (Bbi).
- C3b may become bound to Factor H, another plasma protein. C3bH is then susceptible to an enzyme, Factor I, which converts C3b to an inactive form (C3bi) that can no longer enter the amplification loop.

Alternative pathway activators are generally macromolecules which stabilize the C3bBb enzyme. They may do this by forming a protective surface to which the enzyme adheres, and where it is less susceptible to breakdown. Macromolecules that act as alternative pathway activators are often very long molecules with a highly repetitive structure, seemingly making a highly stabilizing surface.

Bacteria are also known to activate Factor P (properdin), a plasma globulin, such that it changes configuration to provide another stabilizing surface.

Cobra venom factor (CVF) is a very well-known AP activator which works in a somewhat different way. CVF is a molecule with a structure rather similar to C3b. Thus, CVF enters the amplification loop, eventually being responsible for extensive C3 cleavage. However, CVF does not bind to Factor H and cannot be inactivated by Factor I and is therefore not regulated by this loop. The injection of CVF into an animal causes a rapid loss of C3 in plasma as it eventually all gets cleaved by the convertase enzyme.

The alternative pathway can feed into the lytic sequence

C3b, the product of the alternative pathway, can also feed into the common lytic sequence, resulting in lysis of micro-organisms. This happens when a molecule of C3b binds to the alternative pathway convertase to form a new enzyme **C3bBbC3b**, which is a C5 convertase. From this point the two activation pathways merge.

Physiological regulation of complement activation

In its physiological role, careful regulation of complement activity is required to prevent damage to the body, particularly from lytic and inflammatory mediators. Factors H and I are important regulators of C3b production and disposal. Inactive C3b (C3bi) produced by the action of these two proteins is further degraded into smaller fragments, C3dg and C3d, which remain bound to the coated red blood cell. In addition, any C4b that has bound to a red

Table 3.4 *Regulators of complement activity*

Regulator/name	Role
C1INH/C1 inhibitor	Inhibits the action of C1r on C1s and C1s on its substrate
C3bINA/C3b inactivator	Splits cell-bound and fluid phase C3b into two fragments, C3c and C3dg, the latter then being degraded further to yield C3d. This effectively destroys the C5 convertase of both pathways and the independent biological activities of C3b
Carboxypeptidase B	Inhibits the anaphylatoxin activities of C3a and C5a
DAF/decay accelerating factor	Interacts with C4b and C3b so as to allow Factor I to cleave them
Factors H and I	Remove C3b from the amplification loop and convert it to the inactive C3bi

blood cell is degraded to a smaller fragment, C4d, which remains bound. Many antibodies that are potentially lytic to red cells do not proceed to lysis *in vitro* owing to the presence of natural regulators. Therefore, instead of looking for lysis as an end-point of complement activation, the transfusion scientist will look for the presence of cell-bound C3d, using an appropriate antibody.

Some molecules known to regulate complement are shown in Table 3.4. Deficiency of any of these regulators may result in chronic activation of complement.

Complement in transfusion science

A serum containing anti-red blood cell antibodies, particularly of the IgM class, has the potential to cause haemolysis by activation of complement. This is true in transfusion reactions (e.g. anti-A, anti-B) as well as in sera with autoantibodies against red blood cells. Detection of these antibodies is essential. Such antibodies may be detected by haemolysis, using complement, or they may be detected by looking for activated complement proteins coating the surface of red blood cells with which the serum has been incubated.

Establishing complement levels of sera

Occasionally it might be necessary to establish that a serum has normal complement activity. This might be needed, for example, when wishing to detect antibodies to red cells by complement-dependent lysis rather than the more usual agglutination. In such cases, sheep red blood cells coated with a subagglutinating level of anti-sheep red blood cell antibodies are used. Such cells are commonly known as **sensitized sheep red cells**. Serial dilutions of the serum are incubated with sensitized cells and the amount of haemolysis compared with a set of standards to assess the per cent haemolysis, and thus the amount of complement. A serum that has a complement level less than 50% of normal is likely to be unsatisfactory for the detection of complement-fixing antibodies.

Loss of complement activity in sera

Loss of complement can sometimes affect the activity of a serum in demonstrating haemolysis. Factors that diminish complement activity in sera with previously normal complement levels include:

- **Inactivation by heating**: Complement is heat-labile and all complement activity is lost when serum is heated to 56°C for 30 minutes. Heating serum in this way is a standard method for effectively removing complement from a sample. This might be necessary, for example, when trying to demonstrate agglutination, or when standardizing complement levels in sera by first heating and then adding a standard amount of complement from a known source. It should be noted that heating serum at 37°C for 1 hour will also inactivate complement, so care should be taken when thawing frozen sera at this temperature if complement activity is to be retained.

- **Incorrect storage**: Sera should be stored at −20°C to retain complement activity. However, sera that have been exposed to repeated cycles of freezing and thawing, or have been kept at room temperature for long periods, will soon lose their complement activity.

- **Anticoagulants**: Both heparin and EDTA can inhibit complement. EDTA is the worst offender since it is a chelating agent and calcium and magnesium are both required for classical activation. This may present problems when wishing to use plasma, rather than serum, to detect potentially lytic antibodies.

- **Anticomplementary activity**: Some sera may have anticomplementary activity which inhibits the action of complement. Examples of this include sera with raised or abnormal immunoglobulin levels, and sera that have been incorrectly stored and contain a denatured and inactive form of complement known as **complementoid**.

Complement-deficient sera may be restored by the addition of fresh, ABO-compatible serum which has been pooled from a number of samples. Test sera containing anticomplementary activity may be first incubated with red blood cells to allow binding of potentially lytic antibodies, and the cells then washed and fresh pooled serum is added as a source of complement.

Significance of complement binding by anti-red blood cell antibodies

Antibodies to red blood cells may be drug-induced, autoimmune, or antibodies to blood group antigens (see Chapters 5 and 6). All IgM antibodies bind complement efficiently and are therefore potentially highly lytic *in vivo* and *in vitro* (though, as previously mentioned, red blood cells do not usually bind sufficient complement to cause haemolysis *in vitro)*. Examples of red blood cell antibodies that are of the IgM class include anti-A and anti-B and antibodies to the Lewis blood group. In autoimmune haemolytic disorders, antibodies are frequently IgG. Other blood groups in which IgG anti-red cell antibodies predominate include Rhesus, Duffy and Kell. In these cases, haemolysis may or may not result, depending on the IgG subclass, the number of antigenic sites and the affinity of the antibody.

Non-lytic complement-fixing antibodies

Tests for haemolytic antibodies in sera invariably rely on the presence of sufficient antibody to give optimum conditions for lysis of red blood cells following the antigen/antibody reaction. If there is insufficient antibody, as is often the case, the antigen/antibody complex may fix subhaemolytic doses of complement. In such cases the red blood cells become coated with the most stable components of the complement reaction, that is the C3dg and C4d components. These may be detected by using antibodies to these components to stimulate not lysis but haemagglutination. This techniques is discussed in further detail in Chapter 8.

Complement deficiencies

Inherited deficiencies of nearly all the complement components have been found in humans. Deficiencies in C3, Factor H and Factor I lead to increased susceptibility to infection, especially with pyogenic (pus producing) bacteria. Deficiencies in C1, C4 and C2 are associated with the development of **systemic lupus erythematosus**. This is an autoimmune disease in which immune complexes persist in organs such as the kidney and cause inflammatory reactions wherever they are deposited. Deficiencies of the proteins involved in the lytic sequence and Factors D and P lead to increases in susceptibility to *Neisseria meningitidis* and *Neisseria gonorrhoea*. Deficiency of the regulatory protein C1-INH results in hereditary angioneurotic oedema, a condition characterized by episodes of inflammatory swelling in different parts of the body.

Suggested further reading

Engelfreit, C.P. (1992). The immune destruction of red cells. *Transfusion Medicine*, **2**, 1–6.

Frank, M.M. (1994). Complement and kinin. In *Basic And Clinical Immunology*, 8th edn (eds D.P. Stites, A.I. Terr and T.G. Parslow). Stamford: Appleton and Lange.

Law, S.K.A. and Reid, K.B.M. (1995). *Complement*, 2nd edn. Oxford: IRL Press.

Various authors (1991). *Immunology Today*, **12**, 295–326. (This edition is devoted entirely to complement.)

Walport, M.J. and Lachmann, P.J. (1993). Complement. In *Clinical Aspects of Immunology*, 5th edn (eds P.J. Lachmann, D.K. Peters, F.S. Rosen and M.J. Walport), pp. 347–375. Oxford: Blackwell Scientific Press.

Self-assessment questions

1. Which class of antibodies is most efficient at activating complement?
2. Why are there more molecules of complement on a red cell after activation than molecules of the antibody that activated complement?
3. How do complement proteins in plasma appear on the membrane of an antibody-coated red cell?
4. Describe what is meant by an anaphylatoxin. In what way do anaphylatoxins stimulate phagocytosis?
5. Outline one method for assessing complement levels in serum.
6. Describe a method for inactivating complement in serum.
7. Why is blood that has been treated with EDTA to prevent coagulation unsuitable for demonstrating antibody-induced haemolysis?

Key Concepts and Facts

- Complement is the name of a series of proteins which have potent effects on the immune system. When activated, complement causes lysis of cells and can stimulate powerful inflammatory reactions in the body.

- Complement may be activated by some classes of antibody (classical pathway) and has an important role in the removal of immune complexes from the circulation.

- Complement deficiencies are implicated in the development of some immune complex disorders.

- Complement is activated in transfusion reactions and immune haemolytic anaemias.

- Complement is used as a reagent in the laboratory for the detection of potentially haemolytic antibodies in serum.

- The presence of complement on red cells is an indication that antibody has become bound to red cell antigens.

- Some sera may contain anticomplementary activity.

Chapter 4
Basic genetics for blood groups

Learning objectives

After studying this chapter you should confidently be able to:

Define some of the important terms relating to genetics.

Define the nature of DNA and chromosomes.

Describe the gene as a unit of genetic material.

Understand how the Mendelian laws relate to blood group inheritance.

Describe the difference between genotype and phenotype.

Distinguish between types of inheritance, including autosomal, codominant, sex-linked, dominant and recessive.

Discuss the significance and contribution of selected molecular biology techniques.

It is important to understand how blood groups are inherited in order to appreciate the issues involved in typing the blood group of an individual or selecting blood for transfusion purposes. A discussion of the terms involved in genetics (from the Greek word meaning 'to generate') follows. Most of the initial discoveries about how hereditary information is passed down through generations were made by Mendel and were published in 1865. The many discoveries in the first half of the twentieth century concerning the nature of genetic material culminated in the work of Watson and Crick in 1953 who gave a clear insight into the structure of the genetic material deoxyribonucleic acid (DNA) and how inheritance might occur. The explosion of information in the area of molecular biology, which has been central to the development of biology in modern times, has also impacted transfusion science. Indeed modern techniques have been applied to expand our knowledge of the inheritance and nature of blood group antigens, and a wealth of literature is available in this area. This chapter includes a brief overview of traditional genetics, combined with more recent findings relating to blood group systems.

Gregor Mendel was a monk and a mathematician. He was able to show, initially working with pea plants, that all bodily characteristics are inherited as a combination of half from each parent.

DNA and chromosomes

The human body is composed of somatic (body) cells, the nuclei of which each contain 23 pairs of chromosomes: 22 pairs of **autosomes** and one set of sex chromosomes, either XX or XY. The pairs are **homologous**, meaning that they contain the same genes at the same locations. Cells that have the complete set of 23 pairs of chromosomes are called **diploid**. During sexual reproduction, gametes are produced which each have half the number of chromosomes, i.e. they are **haploid.** These cells have one chromosome from each homologous pair and one sex chromosome. Following fertilization, a diploid cell is produced that will give rise to the embryo. Thus, any individual inherits half their chromosomes from the mother and half from the father.

Each chromosome consists of a single strand of DNA. Each DNA molecule is made up of two very long polynucleotide strands running in opposite directions (i.e. they are **antiparallel**). The nucleotides that make up each strand consist of an organic base, a pentose sugar (deoxyribose) and a phosphate group. The nucleotides are joined together by links between the phosphate of one nucleotide and the sugar of the next (the phosphodiester bond). Thus the backbone of each strand is sugar-phosphate-sugar-phosphate etc., while the organic base forms the step of a 'ladder' at right angles to the backbone. The second strand is 'upside down' with respect to the first, bringing the two organic bases close together so that hydrogen bonds can form between them. There are four bases found in DNA: the purines, adenine (A) and guanine (G), and the pyrimidines, thymine (T) and cytosine (C). They 'pair up' in a precise manner: adenine binds to thymine and guanine to cytosine. The double-stranded DNA is then twisted into the characteristic double helix. The sequence of nucleotides in the DNA strand is extremely important since it is a code containing the information required for the synthesis of RNA and protein.

Genes

A gene was defined in 1909 by Johannsen as a hereditary factor that constitutes a single unit of hereditary material and which is part of a chromosome. Genes code for proteins, which in blood group terms means either a polypeptide chain consisting of a specific amino acid sequence or an enzyme, for example a transferase which transfers a sugar on to a substrate. Structurally, genes are segments of the linear DNA strand that makes up the chromosome. The genes are sequences of nucleotides that encode the amino acid sequences of proteins. A sequence of three nucleotides encodes a single amino acid. This triplet sequence is called a **codon.**

There are 64 different ways in which nucleotides containing the four bases can be combined to form triplets. Thus there are more than enough coding sequences to encode the 20 or so different amino acids that are found in proteins. In fact, a single amino acid may be encoded by more than one triplet, for example ACA and ACC both code for threonine. Other triplets are regulatory codons used, for example, for stopping transcription of DNA ('stop' codons). Although the DNA encodes a sequence of amino acids, DNA is first transcribed into RNA in the nucleus which is then 'translated' into protein on the ribosomes in the cytoplasm.

The position of the genes on the chromosome is called the **locus** (plural **loci**). When genes exist in alternative forms at the same locus on homologous chromosomes they are known as **alleles**. The proteins produced by allelic genes may be structurally similar, but even small differences create antigen sites. Some blood group antigens may be amino acid sequences that give rise to a specific blood group. It is interesting to note that the substitution of just one amino acid can result in a different blood group specificity; for some examples see Table 4.1. One example of this in a blood group system is the Rhesus (Rh) group which has multiple alleles (see Chapter 5).

If the genes at a particular locus on homologous chromosomes are the same, then the individual is said to be **homozygous**. The homozygous genes are inherited from both parents, for example the 'C' or 'E' antigens of the Rh system. The antigens that are produced by allelic genes are said to be **antithetical**. For example, antigens within the Kell system that are antithetical are the antigens Kell and Cellano. In blood grouping terms a homozygous individual has more antigen sites for a particular blood group than one who is heterozygous. This effect is seen in the laboratory as giving a stronger agglutination reaction with a corresponding antibody and is referred to as a **dosage effect**. Therefore homozygous individuals exhibit a 'double dose' of the gene product, which in this instance refers to specific blood group antigens, whilst heterozygotes have only a single dose. For examples of blood groups that exhibit dosage effects in laboratory tests, see Chapter 6.

Table 4.1 *Some examples of amino acid substitutions that result in blood group specificity*

Blood group	Antigen	Amino acid	Nucleotide
MNS	M → N	Ser → Leu	C → T
		Gly → Glu	G → A
	S → s	Met → Thr	T → C
Lutheran	Lu^a → Lu^b	His → Arg	A → G
Kidd	Jk^a → Jk^b	Asp → Asn	G → A
Duffy	Fy^a → Fy^b	Gly → Asp	G → A
Rhesus	C → c	Ser → Pro	T → C
		Ile → Leu	A → C
		Ser → Asn	G → A
	E → e	Pro → Ala	C → G

DNA replication and protein synthesis

Before a somatic cell divides, replication of the DNA strand must occur in order to provide the same complement of DNA for the new cells formed by mitosis. This process involves the two DNA strands unwinding (using the enzyme helicase). Each new strand then acts as a template for the formation of a new complementary chain. During protein synthesis DNA partially unwinds and certain portions act as a template for the synthesis of a single-stranded ribonucleic acid (RNA). This messenger RNA (mRNA) is complementary to the DNA region copied and, like all RNA molecules, contains ribose instead of deoxyribose and the pyrimidine uracil instead of thymine.

This process of mRNA production, using DNA as a template, is known as **transcription**. The transcription of DNA to RNA occurs in one direction and transfers the code for DNA to RNA so that the correct sequence of amino acids can be formed. The enzyme DNA polymerase is involved in the process by attaching to the DNA molecule and opening a strand of the double helix. Thus, transcription of DNA occurs as the nascent mRNA peels away from the DNA strand.

This RNA is then transferred from the nucleus to the cytoplasm and attaches to ribosomes, which are the site of protein synthesis. In the cytoplasm, the amino acids, which are free in the cell pool, are brought to the ribosomes by transfer RNA (tRNA). Each amino acid is attached to a specific tRNA containing a sequence of bases which is complementary to the codon and is called the **anticodon**. This tRNA then attaches to mRNA and brings along with it the appropriate amino acid. As the amino acids are joined together by peptide bonds, a polypeptide chain results. This may be further modified within the cell by the addition of carbohydrates and lipids (post-translational modification). Figure 4.1 illustrates the stages involved in protein synthesis that have just been described.

Mutations

As the sequence of bases contains the code for a protein, any change in that sequence, or mutation, will alter the nature of the protein produced. Sometimes mutations or substitutions of single bases within the codon occur spontaneously. The effect of a mutation is a change in the triplet of the codon, which may change the amino acid produced. There are several different types of mutation which produce varying effects on the protein produced.

- **Silent mutations.** A silent mutation may occur because there are several codons for the same amino acid. Thus a change from ACA, which codes for threonine, to ACC, will still result in the code for threonine. Sometimes an amino acid is substituted for

(a) Transcription

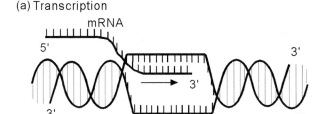

(b) Translation

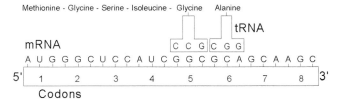

(c) Stages of translation

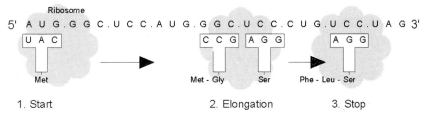

Figure 4.1 *Stages in protein synthesis*

another but this has no evident effect on the phenotype; again this is a siient mutation.

- **Mis-sense mutations.** Substitutions of bases that result in a change in the amino acid sequence may result in the formation of an abnormal protein, and these are **mis-sense mutations.**

- **Frame-shift mutations.** In addition, changes to the codon may be due to insertion or deletion of bases and, in this case, the result is that the reading frame is altered, giving a so-called **frame-shift mutation.** A good example of this is blood group O. Studies have shown that the DNA sequence of the *O* gene is the same as that for *A* gene except that a single base is deleted at the 258 position. The result is still a transferase enzyme but it is non-functional (see Chapter 5).

Other blood group antigens have resulted from DNA mutations; for example, the MNSs blood group system. In this system, the S antigen contains the amino acid methionine, which is encoded by the nucleotide sequence TAC. If the code is altered to TGC, threonine is incorporated instead of methionine giving rise to the

The technique of Southern blotting was first described in 1975 by Dr Edmund Southern of Edinburgh. It uses DNA, which is isolated and cut with restriction enzymes. The fragments are then sorted by size in a gel using electrophoresis where the smaller fragments migrate faster than the larger ones. The fragments are then transferred to a nylon or nitrocellulose membrane and the DNA is denatured into single strands. The sample of DNA is incubated with a probe (a piece of complementary single-stranded DNA) which attaches to the complementary fragment being identified, i.e. a particular gene. The probe is radioactively labelled so that it can be visualized when X-ray film is placed on the membrane and appears as a black band when the film is developed as an autoradiogram. Thus a gene can be identified by determining its size, according to its position, in relation to known fragments of DNA.

s antigen. Gene duplication is shown in the Rhesus system, which has the genes *D* and *CcEe* together on the same chromosome.

The use of molecular biology techniques in recent years has been extremely valuable in developing an understanding of the genetics of blood groups and how they are inherited by individuals. These techniques include DNA typing techniques such as **restriction fragment length polymorphism** analysis (RFLP), the **polymerase chain reaction** (PCR) and the cloning and sequencing of genes. The use of RFLP and PCR has been applied to human leukocyte antigen typing (HLA) for transplant patients (see Chapter 11). **Southern blot analysis** has been used to detect the presence of the gene for blood group O which is otherwise undetectable in the laboratory due to the inactive enzyme produced. The polymerase chain reaction (PCR) is a process of DNA amplification which initially requires a very small amount of DNA. The technique has been applied to the detection of small amounts of viral DNA in blood samples from donors, where the samples are tested for viruses such as human immunodeficiency virus (HIV) and hepatitis B and C viruses to prevent the transmission of disease to recipients of transfused blood. PCR has also been of value in HLA typing of donors and recipients for organ transplantation.

Inheritance of genes

Individuals inherit one set of chromosomes from their mother and one set from their father. The testes in men and the ovaries in women are the sites of production of cells containing a haploid set of chromosomes. These cells are known as **gametes** and are the ova in women and spermatozoa in men. During fertilization of the ovum by a spermatozoa the two haploid nuclei fuse together to form diploid cells. Thus the developing embryo has 23 pairs of chromosomes again. The inheritance of chromosomes and the genes within them is governed by the Mendelian laws of genetics.

Mendelian laws

Mendel derived three laws from the results of his experiments. These are the laws of segregation, independent assortment and dependent assortment. These aspects of inheritance are also relevant in the inheritance of blood groups.

The law of **segregation** refers to the separation of a single pair of genes on homologous chromosomes when they pass to different gametes during the process of meiosis. The law of **independent assortment** states that genes which are not on homologous chromosomes or are situated far apart on homologous chromosomes separate independently and that the complement of chromosomes passed to the sex cell is governed by chance. The genes are not linked together and therefore they separate independently.

Dependent assortment, or **linkage**, states that genes on the same chromosome with gene loci which are close together are inherited together and are said to be 'linked'. As a result, they do not segregate independently and if positioned close together are unlikely to be separated by the process of crossing over which also occurs in meiosis. Examples of linked genes can be seen in the inheritance of the MNSs blood group system which is further described in Chapter 6.

Dominant and recessive genes

When a zygote inherits two identical genes at a particular locus, the zygote is said to be **homozygous** for that gene. When the genes are different, or allelic, the zygote is **heterozygous** for that gene. Allelic genes are said to be **codominant** if both alleles are transcribed and translated such that the products of both genes are found. However, it is often the case that only one allele, the **dominant** gene, is expressed, with the second, non-expressed allele being termed **recessive**. Thus a recessive allele will only be expressed in an individual who is homozygous for that recessive gene, i.e. when no dominant gene is present.

An example of codominant genes is found in the ABO system where the AB blood group results from the inheritance of the two dominant genes, *A* and *B*, one gene originating from the mother and one from the father. In addition, the M and N genes of the MNSs system are codominant. A gene that does not produce a detectable product is known as a silent gene or an **amorph**. This was thought to occur in the ABO system where the 'O' gene appeared to be an amorph but, as stated earlier, it is in fact due to a frame-shift mutation resulting in the wrong codon being formed.

Genotype and phenotype

The terms **genotype** and **phenotype** were described by Johannsen in 1909:

- **Genotype** can be defined as meaning all or a particular part of the genetic constitution of an individual or a cell. In the transfusion laboratory, the genotype of an individual refers to their genetic constitution in relation to a particular blood group. This is often not detectable by the laboratory but may be correctly guessed by investigating the family or by the use of direct genetic techniques. An individual who shows results consistent with blood group A may have the genotype AA or AO depending on the inheritance of the *A* and *O* genes from the parents. It may be important to know the genotype, for example in the case of the father of a baby at risk of developing haemolytic disease of the newborn (see Chapter 7).

> Note that the ultimate gene product is a protein. However, DNA is not translated directly into protein. Instead, the code is first transcribed into mRNA and then translated into a protein in the cytoplasm. An example in blood group terms may be the production of an enzyme or a protein within the cell nucleus.

• **Phenotype** is defined as the observable effects of a gene and thus the phenotype can be deduced from the results of tests in the laboratory. A blood group B individual is phenotypically group B, but it is not known from laboratory tests whether they carry *BB* or *BO* genes, i.e. what their genotype is.

Inheritance of blood groups

The genes responsible for particular blood group antigens may be carried on the autosomal chromosomes or on the sex chromosomes. When they are carried on the sex chromosomes they are linked to the X chromosome. As the genes may also be dominant, codominant or recessive, they can be inherited in a variety of possible ways. Table 4.2 shows some examples.

Most blood groups fall into the category of autosomal dominant or codominant, though X-linked dominant inheritance is occasionally seen, for example in the blood group system Xg^a. The mating of heterozygous individuals may result in a homozygous recessive trait being inherited. For example, H positive parents each of whom are the genotype Hh may produce an offspring who has the genotype hh, and this is the genetic basis of the rare **Bombay phenotype** which is described in Chapter 5. Family pedigrees are sometimes used to trace the inheritance of a particular gene. The term **propositus** (or **proposita**) is used to indicate the individual who is carrying the gene of interest. Pedigree charts use specific symbols to describe the family tree in a diagrammatic form, as shown in Figure 4.2.

Inheritance patterns are also of value when considering population genetics for blood groups, that is, the frequency with which a blood group gene occurs in a given population. Statistics of gene frequencies have been widely used in transfusion science to estimate the most likely genotype for an individual where the results indicate that more than one possibility may exist. This is particularly useful for determining the multiple alleles of the Rhesus system and is referred to in more detail in Chapter 5. A knowledge of the population frequencies of blood groups is also useful in the screening of compatible blood for transfusion to a patient. If the patient is known to possess a number of different antibodies to blood groups, an increased number of units of donor blood must be screened before compatible blood may be selected.

The **Hardy–Weinberg formula** has been used to determine the frequency of a gene in a population. Hardy was a mathematician and Weinberg a physician, who together addressed the possible reason why a recessive trait would not eventually be lost from a population. They produced a mathematical formula, based on a binomial equation, which requires certain conditions for its basis. These include a large population with random mating, no mutations and no migration. Whilst these are not entirely true of the human population, the formula has nevertheless been of use in determining population genetics.

Table 4.2 *Some examples of blood group antigen inheritance patterns*

Chromosome	Inheritance	Antigen
Autosomal	Dominant	A, B
Autosomal	Codominant	AB, MN
X-linked	Dominant	Xg^a, Xg^k

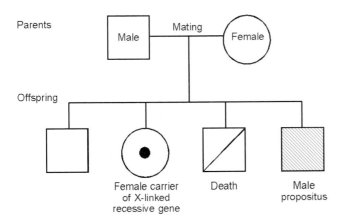

Figure 4.2 *Example of a pedigree chart illustrating symbols used*

Suggested further reading

Bryant, N.J. (1994). *An Introduction to Immunohematology*. Philadelphia: W.B. Saunders Company.

Moulds, J.M. (1994). Basic genetics. In *Modern Blood Banking and Transfusion Practices* (ed. D.M. Harmening). Philadelphia: F.A. Davis Company.

Passarge, E. (1995). *Color Atlas of Genetics*. New York: Georg Thieme Verlag.

Self-assessment questions

1. What is a codon?
2. Define the term 'allele'.
3. List the organic bases of DNA.
4. What type of inheritance would show a gene appearing in each generation with equal frequency between the sexes?
5. Differentiate between independent assortment and dependent assortment of genetic material (genes).
6. What is the role of tRNA in protein synthesis?
7. Describe three types of genetic mutation.

Key Concepts and Facts

- The inheritance of genes was first described by Gregor Mendel and has since been applied to the inheritance of blood group systems.

- Normal diploid cells contain 23 pairs of chromosomes whilst haploid cells, i.e. the gametes, contain 23 single chromosomes.

- The structure of DNA consists of nucleotides formed from an organic base, a pentose sugar and a phosphate group.

- The organic bases of DNA are adenine, guanine, cytosine and thymine, and the sequence of bases forms the genetic code.

- A gene is a single unit of hereditary material located on a chromosome. It consists of sequences of DNA coding for proteins.

- The genetic code is a triplet one in which the sequence of three nucleotides encodes a single amino acid.

- Protein synthesis results from the transcription of the genetic code and its translation into a protein.

- Blood group systems are inherited via dominant, recessive or codominant genes, which are usually autosomal.

- The Mendelian laws of segregation, and dependent and independent assortment are also seen in the genetics of blood group systems.

- The genotype and phenotype of the blood group of an individual may be established using inheritance patterns and population frequencies and by laboratory procedures, including the increasing use of molecular biology techniques.

Chapter 5

Introduction to the ABO and Rhesus blood group systems

Learning objectives

After studying this chapter you should confidently be able to:

Discuss the historical aspects of the ABO and Rhesus systems.

Outline the cellular and molecular bases of the ABO and Rhesus systems.

Describe the subgroups of A and B.

Describe the genetics of the ABO and Rhesus systems.

Describe the roles of the secretor and *H* genes.

Describe the frequency of the ABO and Rhesus types in selected populations.

The ABO and Rh blood groups will be considered in detail in this chapter because of their importance in blood transfusion. Other blood group systems, which will be described in the following chapter, include: Lewis, P, Ii, Kidd, Kell, Duffy, Lutheran and MNSs.

The following conventions have been adopted throughout this book:

- Existing 'popular' terminology is used for blood systems and antigens.
- Superscripts and subscripts are used where appropriate.
- The presence or absence of antigens is indicated by a plus or minus sign, respectively.
- Genes are written in italics.
- Antibodies are written in terms of their antigen notation, with the prefix 'anti-'.
- International Society of Blood Transfusion (ISBT) notations are also included.

The earliest reports of blood transfusions in modern times appeared

Karl Landsteiner was a remote, austere man who was awarded the Nobel prize in medicine in 1930 for his discovery of blood groups. His work in the finding of red cell 'agglutinogens' and serum 'agglutinins' led to the discovery of the ABO system.

Landsteiner was working at the Institute of Pathological Anatomy in Vienna, Austria, in 1900 when he conducted his experiment on six men from his laboratory. These included four researchers, an unknown man labelled 'Zar' and Karl Landsteiner himself. Blood was taken from each and separated into cells and serum by allowing it to clot. The red cells were diluted in saline to a suspension of 5% concentration and each serum placed in a test tube with each sample of red cells. This gave 36 results which could either show agglutination or remain unagglutinated. The red cells of two samples, from Landsteiner and another colleague, showed no agglutination with any of the other sera, but their sera did agglutinate the red cells of the other four. The results of the other four samples fell into two groups of two, each showing reciprocal agglutination patterns. It was also noted that no cell sample was agglutinated by its own serum. The two patterns of agglutination were called A and B, respectively, and the serum with both agglutinins was initially called C. Thus the ABO system was first described. It is interesting to note, considering the frequency of occurrence of the ABO groups in the German population at the time, that the chance of Landsteiner testing six men at random and finding two of each blood group (A, B and O) is 0.031! However, Landsteiner was to become the founder of immunochemistry and immunohaematology.

in the seventeenth century. One of the first successful transfusions of human blood took place in 1825 when a woman who lost blood in labour was revived using blood donated by her husband. However, blood transfusion was often fatal until the experiments by Landsteiner in 1900 gave evidence of the ABO blood group system.

The ABO blood group system (ISBT 001, symbol ABO)

The ABO system consists of the blood groups A, B, AB and O, with further subdivisions of A and B. The nomenclature is based on the presence of oligosaccharide substances, which act as blood group antigens due to their ability to bind to antibodies. These antigens can be detected on red blood cells and many other body cells. They are also present in body fluids. Testing of blood for transfusion to determine the ABO group is imperative in order to prevent blood transfusion reactions in a patient, the result of which may be fatal.

Landsteiner discovered three of the four blood groups in the ABO system in 1900. The year 1900 was also the year in which Gregor Mendel's laws of heredity were rediscovered, having first been proposed in 1895. Subsequent discoveries in the area of blood groups allowed for much progress in genetic knowledge. Landsteiner took blood from six of his colleagues, allowed it to clot, and then tested each serum against the red cells of each of the other samples. He noted that the results either showed agglutination between the red cells and sera or no agglutination. Furthermore, the results of agglutinated samples fell into two different patterns. Thus he proposed that two antigens on the red cells were involved, which he called A and B. Those cells which had not agglutinated must lack these antigens and were therefore designated O (for zero). Landsteiner's law states that the presence of the antigen on the cells implies the absence of the corresponding antibody in the serum and the presence of the opposite antibody. Thus, group O individuals would have antibodies to both A and B antigens. A fourth blood group in which both antigens were detectable was described in 1902 by von DeCastello and Sturli. This was called AB and neither antibody A nor B could be detected in the serum of these individuals. Table 5.1 shows the antigens and antibodies of the ABO system and Table 5.2 shows the results of ABO grouping using known antisera and red cells.

The biochemical nature of the A and B antigens

The A and B antigens are defined by specific **sugars** attached to a chain of **oligosaccharides** known as the **'precursor substance'**. This precursor substance protrudes from the red cell membrane and is attached to **glycolipids** which form part of the red blood cell

Table 5.1   *The red cell antigens and serum antibodies of the ABO system*

Red cell antigens	Serum antibodies	Blood group
Antigen A	Antibody B	A
Antigen B	Antibody A	B
Neither A nor B	Antibodies A and B	O
Both A and B	Neither A nor B antibodies	AB

NB The blood group is always designated by the antigens on the red cells. The antigens are detectable on foetal red blood cells and throughout life.

Table 5.2   *Results of ABO blood grouping using known antisera and red cells*

Patient red cell sample	Agglutination using anti-A	Agglutination using anti-B	Blood group
1	+	Negative	A
2	Negative	+	B
3	+	+	AB
4	Negative	Negative	O

Patient serum sample	Agglutination using A cells	Agglutination using B cells	Blood group
1	Negative	+	A
2	+	Negative	B
3	Negative	Negative	AB
4	+	+	O

membrane structure. Before these sugars can be attached to the precursor chain, it is necessary that the individual is genetically able to attach **L-fucose**, which is known as **H substance**, to the precursor chain.

The sugars involved in the ABO system are L-fucose (H determining sugar), N-acetylgalactosamine (A determining sugar) and D-galactose (B determining sugar). Figure 5.1 illustrates a three-dimensional, computer generated model of the sugars showing their spatial arrangement.

The blood group determining sugars are added in the Golgi apparatus of the cells. Enzymes are required for the attachment of the sugars to the precursor chain. These enzymes are glycosyl transferases, i.e. they transfer a sugar from one molecule to another. The production of these transferases is dependent on the presence of the gene specific for their formation.

Oligosaccharides are carbohydrate polymers of between 3 and 20 sugar residues. They attach by covalent bonds to lipid and protein, often forming a branched structure of side chains which allows for a great variety of shapes and sizes due to the many possibilities for linking within the chains. This results in a large number of different blood groups as each configuration appears to be different. This evokes an antibody-producing response in a person not already carrying that 'antigen' on their red blood cells.

Ceramides are fatty acids joined to sphingosine by an amide linkage.

Gangliosides are also important in blood group antigen structures. These differ from cerebrosides in that their oligosaccharide head group contains one to four **sialic acid** residues. These have a negative charge at pH 7 so that the red cell surface has an overall negative charge.

Figure 5.1 *Computer generated models of the terminal portion of A, B and O antigens. (Courtesy of C.A. Smith, Department of Biological Sciences, Manchester Metropolitan University)*

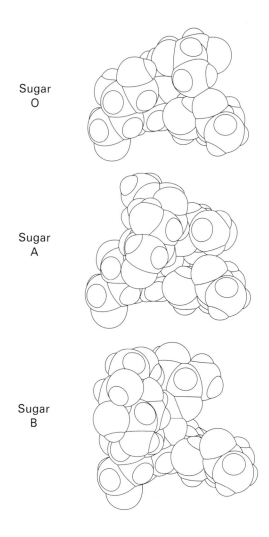

Sugar
O

Sugar
A

Sugar
B

Genes involved in the ABO system

The genes responsible for the enzyme production have been located on chromosome 6. The *H* gene codes for the production of the enzyme **L-fucosyl transferase**, which transfers the sugar L-fucose (Fuc) to the terminal sugar of the precursor chain, galactose. This is known as the **H** structure and is the structure found in individuals of the blood group O. In addition, the *Z* gene regulates the production of H antigen on red cells. If the *Z* gene is absent, i.e. the person is *zz*, no H antigen is produced (a rare occurrence). The *A* gene encodes for the production of N-**acetylgalactosaminyl transferase**, which transfers N-acetylgalactosamine (GalNAc) to the H structure, giving the A antigen which is found on the red cells of blood group A individuals. The *B* gene encodes **D-galactosyl transferase** which transfers D-galactose (Gal) to the H structure, resulting in blood group B. However, if both *A* and *B* genes are present on the chromosome, both sugars are attached to

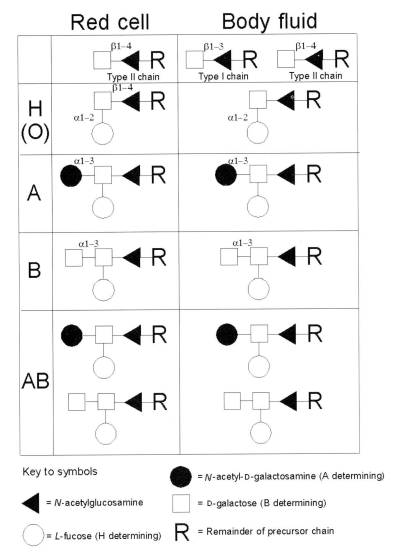

Figure 5.2 *Biochemical basis of ABO blood group system*

the H structure in a random way, as is found on the red cells of blood group AB individuals.

The nature and sequence of the sugars is important in conferring antigenicity, and the type of glycosidic bond joining the sugars together is also important. The precursor substance may be formed by linkage of the sugars to each other at different positions. Type 1 chains exhibit α1–3 linkage in which the carbon at position one of galactose is attached to the carbon at position three of N-acetylglucosamine in the precursor substance. Type 2 chains show a β1–4 linkage. L-Fucose is attached to the precursor substance by α1–2 linkage. Figure 5.2 shows the biochemical basis of the structures of the A, B and H antigens, illustrating the sugars involved and the way in which they are attached to each other.

The secretor gene

The ABH antigens may also be secreted into the body fluids, such as sweat, saliva, semen, breast milk, tears and digestive juices, with the exception of cerebrospinal fluid due to the blood–brain barrier. These antigens are widely distributed on a range of cells including white blood cells (leukocytes), platelets, epithelial cells, spermatozoa and gastric mucosal cells. In embryonic development these are all cells derived from the endoderm.

In order that the antigens may be secreted into body fluids the individual must carry the gene which confers 'secretor status', i.e. the secretor gene. Endodermically derived tissues have H antigen generated by α2-L-fucosyl transferase. This is the enzyme encoded by the secretor gene. It acts on the terminal galactose of the type 1 precursor chain (the secreted ABH glycoprotein substances are attached by both type 1 and 2 linkages, whereas the ABH sugars are attached by type 1 linkage only). Non-secretor individuals have little or no expression of ABO blood group antigens in body fluids because they lack α2-L-fucosyl transferase and so cannot transfer L-fucose. Secretor status may be inherited in the homozygous state *Se/Se*, or heterozygous *Se/se*. Approximately 75% of the Caucasian population are secretors of blood group substances. The other 25% are homozygous non-secretors with *se/se* status. Secretor status can be detected by testing the saliva for the presence of A or B blood group substances and H substance. Thus group A individuals will secrete A and H substances, group B will have B and H substances and AB individuals will have A, B and H substances in their saliva. Group O individuals secrete only H substance.

The H gene and the Bombay blood groups

The presence and importance of the *H* gene was demonstrated by a family study described by Bhende in 1952. This study showed that the presence of the *H* gene, inherited either as the homozygous form *HH* or heterozygous *Hh*, is necessary for the conversion of the oligosaccharide precursor substance to H substance, i.e. the addition of L-fucose to the precursor chain. Thus individuals who are genotype *hh* are unable to produce A and B antigens (i.e. sugars) even though they have the gene for A or B transferases. Consequently, when tested in the laboratory, the red blood cells give the agglutination reaction of group O although the serum contains anti-A, anti-B and anti-H. This is known as a 'Bombay blood group' and such individuals are denoted as being blood group OhA, OhB or Oh. Whilst this is a rare group, it is important to detect this blood type in the laboratory as blood from a Bombay phenotype is not compatible with other ABO groups and such an individual needs to be transfused with Bombay type blood.

Table 5.3 *ABO phenotypes and genotypes*

Phenotype	Possible genotype
A_1	A_1A_1 or A_1A_2 or A_1O
A_2	A_2A_2 or A_2O
B	BB or BO
O	OO
A_1B	A_1B
A_2B	A_2B

Inheritance of the ABO groups

In 1910 von Dungern and Hirzfeld proved that the ABO blood groups were inherited and three allelic genes, designated *A*, *B* and *O*, were proposed by Bernstein in 1924. Each individual inherits two genes, one from each parent. The A antigen was later found to consist of two forms, A_1 and A. Individuals with red blood cells expressing both A_1 and A antigens are termed blood group A_1 whilst those with only the one form of A antigen are typed as A_2. The difference between A_1 and A antigens is due to the quantity of antigen sites and to differences in the antigens themselves.

The four allelic genes could give rise to six possible phenotypes: A_1, A_2, B, O, A_1B and A_2B. The *A* and *B* genes are codominant, so that they are expressed if they are present on the chromosome. Furthermore, the *A* gene is dominant over *O*, which is an amorph (i.e. a gene which has no detectable product). The phenotype is the detectable blood group and the genotype refers to the genetic information upon which the phenotype is based (see Chapter 4). Table 5.3 illustrates the phenotypes and genotypes of the ABO blood group system.

Subgroups of A and B

The number of antigen sites on the membrane of the red blood cell has led to the establishing of subgroups. The majority of blood group A individuals belong to blood group A_1. The presence of the A_1 antigen can be detected using a **plant lectin** specific to the A_1 antigen. This has been extracted from the seeds of the plant *Dolichos biflorus* and is available commercially. These individuals show a weak agglutination when incubated with anti-A. Subgroups A_3 and A_4 (also called A_x) have much less A antigen present on the cells, sometimes called diminished expression. Other weak subgroups are A_y and A_{end}. The latter has an absence of transferase activity. Blood group B also contains some weaker forms, identified as B_3, B_w, B_x and B_m, which are rarely seen in Caucasian populations.

Table 5.4 *Distribution of ABO phenotypes in various populations*

Phenotype	Caucasian (%)	Black (%)	Oriental (%)	Indian (%)	Australian aborigine (%)
O	44	49	43	22	44
A_1	34	19	27	22	56
A_2	10	8	2	2	0
B	9	19	25	38	0
A_1B	3	3	5	15	0

Population distribution of ABO groups

The ABO blood groups are distributed differently in various populations and this may be determined by inheritance and population mobility. It is generally accepted in the United Kingdom that blood group O is the most common, although in the north-west of England, transfusion centres have found it to be blood group A. The United States population may be broadly considered in terms of Western European descent, in which 'A' is the most common (45%) followed by 'O' (43%), and African descent, in which 50% of the population is blood group O, 29% blood group A and 17% blood group B. In each case group AB is rare, at approximately 4%. Thus the distribution of ABO phenotypes varies in different populations throughout the world (see Table 5.4).

The distribution of ABO determining antigens

The number of antigens on red cells varies between different ABO groups and at different stages of the red blood cell development as the cell membrane is becoming established. Also the cells obtainable from the umbilical cord of a newborn infant have significantly fewer antigen sites for A, B and H expressed on their surface than the red cells from an adult. It is important to be aware of this in the laboratory detection of blood groups, as fewer antigen sites result in a weaker agglutination reaction. The number of antigens gradually increases from foetal life until adolescence. A comparison of antigen site numbers can be seen in Table 5.5.

Molecular biology techniques and the ABO antigens

Knowledge of the molecules that make up the blood groups has been expanding in recent years due to advances in biochemical and molecular experimental techniques. The molecular basis of the ABO antigens has been studied in particular. The genes for the glycosyl transferases have now been cloned using molecular tech-

Table 5.5   *Number of A, B and H antigens on red blood cells*

Cell type	Number of A antigen sites
A_1 adult	800 000–1 000 000
A_2 adult	250 000
A_3 adult	35 000
A_4 adult	4800
A_1 cord	250 000–300 000
A_1B adult	460 000–850 000
A_2B adult	140 000

Cell type	Number of B antigen sites
B adult	750 000
B cord	200 000–300 000
A_1B adult	430 000

Cell type	Number of H antigen sites
O adult	1 700 000
O cord	325 000
AB cord	70 000

niques. The molecular basis of the silent phenotypes such as the O blood group, non-secretors and Bombay blood groups has been clarified.

It is becoming possible to classify blood group antigens into categories which relate to cellular function, such as transporters and channels, adhesion molecules, receptors and ligands, enzymes and structural proteins. The molecular basis of ABH expression was established by the cDNA cloning of the glycosyl transferase for blood group A. Thus the structures of the enzymes have been established. The difference between the A and B transferases is due to the substitution of four amino acids (Arg176Gly, Gly235Ser, Leu266Met, Gly268Ala).

Blood group O phenotypes are the result of three different alleles. The prototype O^1 is due to a single base deletion at codon 87 in the transferase gene and this causes a **frame-shift mutation**. The result is that an inactive polypeptide chain consisting of 117 amino acids is produced. It is thought that 56% of blood group O individuals belong to this type, whilst 40% are of the O^{1var} type which also has the base deletion but in addition has five silent base substitutions in the transferase gene. A rare allele (4%), designated O^2, is a **missense mutation** resulting in an enzymatically inactive transferase.

ABO blood group antibodies

These antibodies are present in the sera of healthy adults and older children. The antibodies are formed when the corresponding antigen is absent – a phenomenon sometimes known as Landsteiner's law. Thus, antibody A (anti-A) is found in the sera of groups B and O and anti-B is found in groups A and O. If both A and B antigens are present on the red cells, as in group AB, no antibodies are formed, and if neither A nor B antigens are present, as in group O, both anti-A and anti-B are formed. Anti-A_1 is found in the sera of groups B and O as a component of anti-A_1, i.e. anti-A is a mixture of anti-A and anti-A_1. Anti-A_1 is also found in the sera of approximately 2% of group A adults and 25% of group A_2B adults. Also found in the sera of group A_1, A_1B and B adults is anti-H. Anti-H is always found in the sera of individuals who carry the rare Bombay blood type.

The antibodies are usually of the IgM class though they may occur as a mixture of IgM, IgG and Ig A. They are formed at 3–6 months of age, gradually increasing in titre to peak at age 5–10 years. After this the levels slowly decline as age increases and they may be barely detectable in older people. Although they are called 'naturally occurring' antibodies, they result from the stimulus of non-pathogenic micro-organisms associated with ingested food. The antibodies react optimally with their corresponding antigens at room temperature (approximately 16–22°C). Thus they are considered to be 'cold agglutinins'. They may also be able to bind complement at 37°C and in this event would be of concern when transfused to a patient. In addition, anti-A and anti-B may occur as immune IgG antibodies if their production is stimulated by pregnancy or blood transfusion. These antibodies readily bind complement and may cause haemolysis of the patient's red cells at 37°C. Thus they are considered to be the most clinically significant of all the blood group antibodies. A transfusion of ABO incompatible blood, meaning the transfusion of group A blood to group O or group B patients or group B blood to group O or A patients, is often fatal. Blood group O is sometimes transfused in emergencies to patients who are group A or B. This may also be fatal if the donor blood contains a high titre of anti-A or anti-B haemolysins (i.e. antibodies which cause haemolysis of red cells). Immune anti-A and anti-B may also cause haemolytic disease of the newborn.

The Rhesus system (ISBT 004, symbol RH)

The Rhesus system was discovered in 1940 by Landsteiner and Wiener. They injected rabbits and guinea pigs with the red cells from Macacus rhesus monkeys and the resulting antibody reacted with the red cells of 85% of New York blood donors. Those who reacted were said to have the Rhesus factor and were Rhesus positive, while those that did not react lacked the Rhesus factor and were Rhesus negative. The terms Rhesus positive or Rh positive and Rhesus negative or Rh negative are still used today, especially by clinical staff, to describe what we now know as Rh D positive and Rh D negative.

By 1945 the original Rh factor had been renamed D and four more Rh antigens discovered. These were the antithetical antigens C and c, and E and e (for further information about antithetical genes, see Chapter 4). There are now 45 antigens in the Rh system but D, C, c, E and e are the most commonly identified and the most significant in blood transfusion. The Rh antigens are expressed on polypeptides. The Rh polypeptides span the red cell membrane exposing six extracellular loops on which are expressed the Rh antigens. These polypeptides are associated in the membrane with an Rh glycoprotein to form tetramers (two Rh polypeptides and two Rh glycoproteins), which form the Rh core complex. The Rh glycoprotein is essential for the formation of this Rh core complex. Defects in its structural gene result in the Rh_{null} phenotype, in which no Rh antigens are expressed. Red cell defects seen in the Rh_{null} phenotype include abnormal cation transport across the red cell membrane and red cell morphological abnormalities. The function of the Rh polypeptide is not known for certain, but it seems likely that it is involved in cation transport across the red cell membrane. The Rh antigens are well developed before birth, being detectable in the 6-week-old foetus. They are fully expressed on cord blood cells. Rh antigens have not been demonstrated on leukocytes and platelets, or found in saliva or amniotic fluid.

> In 1939, Levine and Stetson had described an antibody in a mother who had recently had a stillborn foetus. The antibody caused a haemolytic transfusion reaction when she was transfused with ABO compatible blood from her husband. They suggested that the antibody had been produced in response to an antigen carried by the foetus which had been inherited from the father. This antibody was subsequently shown to have the same reaction pattern as Landsteiner and Wiener's anti-Rh, and so Rh haemolytic disease of the newborn was described for the first time.

Inheritance and nomenclature of the Rh system

Two genetic systems were originally proposed to explain the relationships and inheritance of these five original Rh antigens. In the US, Wiener proposed a system comprising a single locus producing factors he called agglutinogens that could express multiple antigens. In the UK, Fisher and Race proposed a system of three closely linked loci for D/d, C/c and E/e, each gene coding for the production of a single antigen. Thus the antigens C and c were the products of the codominant alleles C and c. Antigens E and e were the products of the codominant alleles E and e. The D antigen was the product of the D gene and the proposed allelic gene d was considered an amorph as no d antigen or anti-d antibody was ever discovered. Fisher also postulated that the order of the genes on a chromosome was DCE, and it has become common practice to refer to them in this order.

Considerable work was carried out by many investigators to elucidate the Rh system because of its clinical significance. As new Rh antigens and phenotypes were discovered it became apparent that neither Wiener's nor Fisher's system could explain every new finding. However, Fisher's system of three closely linked loci was the most complete and allowed the deduction of phenotypes of offspring from different mating types. Fisher's shorthand notation

> In 1962, Rosenfield and colleagues proposed a numerical system for describing the Rhesus antigens. This system was free from the genetic implications of either Wiener's or Fisher's systems, as it merely recorded the observed serological reactions. The (known) Rh antigens were numbered from 1 (for D) to 24, in order of discovery. The numbering of Rh antigens has now reached 51 although, because of obsolete forms, there are now 45 antigens in the system.

> Race and Sanger showed their early Rh typing results to Fisher in the Bun Shop (a Cambridge pub). The first outline of his DCE theory, on 22 June 1944, was described on a pub beer mat.

The Rh D antigen is the most immunogenic of all the protein antigens. It has been reported that as many as 80% of Rh D negative individuals receiving a transfusion of Rh D positive red cells will produce anti-D antibody. Also, as many as 16% of Rh D negative mothers exposed to a foeto-maternal haemorrhage from an Rh D positive foetus will produce anti-D antibody. Despite the success of anti-D prophylaxis, anti-D is still the most common cause of clinically significant haemolytic disease of the newborn.

was also very convenient for communicating information regarding phenotypes and genotypes.

It has now been shown by modern molecular biology techniques that neither of these earlier systems was completely correct and that, in fact, the Rh system is controlled by two closely linked loci. One carries the gene for the Rh D polypeptide and is known as the *RHD* locus. The other carries the genes for the CcEe polypeptide and is known as the *RHCE* locus.

Despite the new evidence concerning the genetics and biochemistry of the Rh system, Fisher's model and shorthand notation continue to be a convenient way to explain and communicate Rh phenotypes and genotypes. For this reason it is outlined below in a little more detail.

Fisher's DCE system

In the Fisher model, three pairs of closely linked alleles (now known to be two pairs) allow for eight possible haplotype arrangements of Rh genes on a chromosome (see Figure 5.3). This is shown in Table 5.6 and the possible genotypes are shown in Table 5.7.

Each set of three alleles is inherited together due to the close linkage of the loci. Each may be paired with itself or any other arrangement, giving 36 possible genotypes. The eight most common ones are listed in Table 5.7 along with their frequencies. It should be noted that the vast majority of Rh D negative individuals are dce/

Table 5.6   *Fisher's model of haplotypes and their frequency*

Haplotype	Shorthand notation	Approx. frequency in Whites (%)	Haplotype	Shorthand notation	Approx. frequency in Whites (%)
DCe	R_1	41	dCe	r′	1
DcE	R_2	14	dcE	r″	1
Dce	R_0	3	dce	r	39
DCE	R_Z	<1	dCE	r^Y	<1
Rh D positive			Rh D negative		

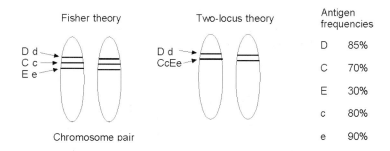

Figure 5.3 *Suggested gene locations for the Fisher and two-locus theories*

Table 5.7 *Fisher's model of genotypes and their frequency*

Genotype	Shorthand notation	Approx. frequency (%)	Genotype	Shorthand notation	Approx. frequency (%)
DCe/dce	R_1r	33	dce/dce	rr	15
DcE/dce	R_2r	11			
Dce/dce	R_0r	2			
DCe/DCe	R_1R_1	18			
DcE/DcE	R_2R_2	2			
DCe/DcE	R_1R_2	14			
DCe/Dce	R_1R_0	2			
All other combinations	<1%		All other combinations < 1%		
Rh D positive			Rh D negative		

Table 5.8 *Examples of the frequency of the D antigen in various populations*

	Rh D positive (%)	Rh D negative (%)
Europe	83	17
West Africa	97	3
India	90	10
Japan	99.7	0.3
China	93	7

dce (rr) and therefore capable of being immunized by exposure to C+ and E+ red cells.

It is vital that students are familiar with the Fisher shorthand notations and their implied genotypes. It is with these shorthand expressions that blood transfusion laboratory workers communicate Rh system information on a day to day basis.

Two-locus model

In this model, suggested by Tippett in 1986, the Rh system is controlled by two closely linked loci (see Figures 5.4–5.6). The *RHD* locus carries the gene for the RHD polypeptide which expresses all the D antigen epitopes. The *RHCE* locus carries the genes for the RHCE polypeptide which expresses both the C/c and E/e antigens. The genes that encode the C/c and E/e antigens are codominant alleles, and the Rh genes are located on chromosome 1.

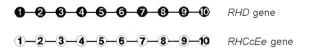

Figure 5.4 *Diagrammatic representation of the RHD and RHCE genes. Each gene is made up of 10 exons, which are shown numbered 1 to 10*

Figure 5.5 *Diagrammatic representation of Rh D positive and Rh D negative gene arrangements*

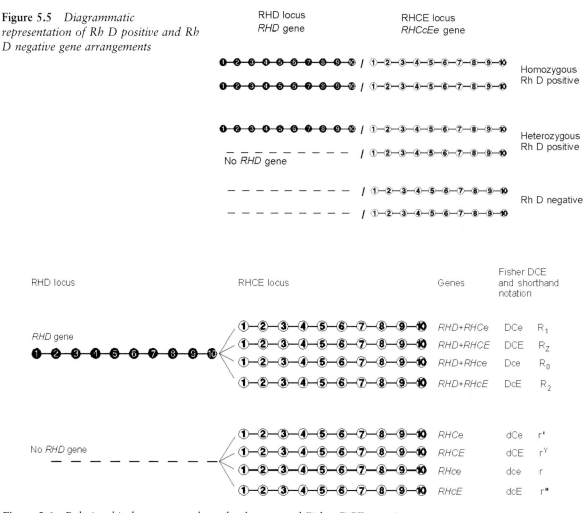

Figure 5.6 *Relationship between two-locus haplotypes and Fisher DCE notation*

The *RHD* and *RHCE* loci are very similar, each comprising 10 exons. The corresponding polypeptides are therefore very similar, differing only at 36 of the 417 amino acid residues in each polypeptide. The C/c antigen polymorphism appears to be associated with four amino acid exchanges, whereas the E/e polymorphism is associated with a single amino acid exchange (see Table 5.9). Transfer of exons between *RHD* and *RHCE* loci, and vice versa, is known to occur. This causes variations in epitope expression and hence antigen expression. Figures 5.7 and 5.8 depict the location of the RHD and RHCE polypeptide chains in the red cell membrane. It can be seen that they are transmembrane proteins.

Expression of Rh epitopes is dependent on the sequence and shape of the amino acids within the polypeptide chain, i.e. conformation. Changes in amino acid sequences or exchange of exons can not only lead to the expression of new epitopes but can also

Table 5.9 *Amino acids (AA) involved in the C/c and E/e polymorphisms*

Antigen expressed		AA position	Exon
C	c		
Cysteine	Tryptophan	16	1
Isoleucine	Leucine	60	2
Serine	Asparagine	68	2
Serine	Proline	103*	2

Antigen expressed		AA position	Exon
E	e		
Proline	Alanine	226	5

* This amino acid is located on the second external loop and is considered crucial for C/c expression.

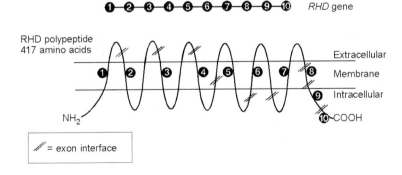

Figure 5.7 *Diagram of the RHD polypeptide chain within the red cell membrane*

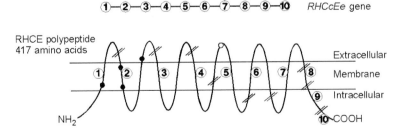

Figure 5.8 *Diagram of the RHCE polypeptide*

cause conformational changes which may affect the expression of other epitopes.

Epitopes are the recognition sites of antibodies and thus each antibody has a specific epitope. Polyclonal antibodies produced in humans are usually a mixture of antibodies to several related epitopes or groups of epitopes. Monoclonal antibodies, which are used in laboratory testing for Rh status, are more usually specific for a single epitope or group of epitopes (see Chapter 2). The RHD and RHCE polypeptides may be thought of as expressing many different epitopes which together express the antigens of the Rh system.

Qualitative differences in Rh antigens

The Rh D antigen is now considered to be made up of at least 30 different epitopes. Monoclonal antibodies have been produced whose reaction patterns reveal these epitopes. Rare individuals who lack certain epitopes are known as **partial D** and may be stimulated to produce antibodies to the missing epitopes by transfusion or pregnancy.

This partial D state may arise from the replacement of an exon segment from *RHD* by an equivalent segment from *RHCE*, creating a hybrid *RHD-CE-D* gene, or as the result of point mutation within RHD. This is illustrated in Figure 5.9. The replacement of several exon segments from *RHD* with the equivalent segments from *RHCE* can destroy the ability to produce D antigen altogether, so that the individual only expresses the C/c and E/e antigens and serologically appears as Rh D negative although they do possess an *RHD* gene.

The G antigen

The G antigen is usually only detected on red cells expressing D antigen or C antigen or both. Its expression appears to be dependent on amino acid sequences derived from exon 2 of the *RHD* gene. Anti-G has been implicated in haemolytic disease of the newborn. The presence of the G antigen explains the not uncommon observation that some non-transfused, pregnant women apparently produce anti-C + D antibody even though the father of their foetus is found to be C negative. In such cases the father has been found to have passed an R_2 chromosome (DcE) to the foetus. The G antigen would also be expressed by this gene arrangement. So the mother has actually been immunized to produce anti-D and anti-G rather than anti-D and anti-C.

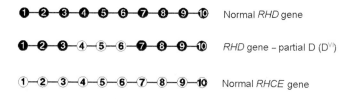

Figure 5.9   Diagram showing how exon exchange gives rise to a partial D gene

Compound antigens

Not unexpectedly, given that the CcEe antigens are produced by the same gene, antibodies have been described which only react with **compound antigens** that are produced by the same gene. For example, the antibody produced in response to the ce compound antigen is anti-ce (it is also known as anti-f). This antibody will only react with cells expressing both c and e antigens derived from the same gene. This means that anti-ce will react with dce (r) or Dce (R_0) red cells but not with DCe/DcE (R_1R_2) cells where the c and e antigens have been produced by different genes. Other examples of compound antigens with corresponding antibodies are cE, CE and Ce.

Quantitative differences in Rh antigens

Antigen dosage

This is the property displayed when antibodies give stronger reactions in laboratory tests with red cells showing homozygous expression of the corresponding antigen than with heterozygotes. The dosage effect when the D antigen is reacted with anti-D is not very noticeable as there is considerable overlap in the number of Rh D sites between the various genotypes. Table 5.10 gives typical examples of D antigen site numbers for various genotypes and clearly indicates the overlapping of D antigen expression between genotypes.

The replacement of several exon segments from the *RHCE* gene with the equivalent segments from the *RHD* gene can destroy the ability to produce C/c and E/e antigens. Such individuals may only express the D antigen and their phenotype is written as D−−. These individuals express much more D antigen on their red cells than

In 1953, Wiener proposed that the Rh D antigen was a mosaic made up of four parts, which he termed Rh^A, Rh^B, Rh^C and Rh^D. Rare individuals who lack part of this mosaic (partial D) may produce immune anti-D specific for the epitopes they lack. In the 1960s, Tippett identified seven D categories by cross-testing the cells and sera of Rh D positive individuals with anti-D in their serum. These D categories were designated using superscript Roman numerals I to VII, e.g. category D^{III}, category D^{VI}. Some of the categories were also subdivided. Further partial D types have been identified by their reaction patterns with monoclonal anti-D.

There has been no real systematic approach to naming these partial D types. By 1993 there was a nine epitope model for Rh D and by 1995 a 30 epitope model. It is now most usual to see partial D types written as their D category (or name if not in a category) together with the epitopes they express and/or lack in either the nine or 30 epitope model or both. This can make for difficult reading for students, and for even more difficult conversation.

Table 5.10 *The distribution of antigens on red cells*

Group	Number of antigen sites
DCe/dce (R_1r)	D sites: 9900–14 600
Dce/dce (R_0r)	D sites: 12 000–20 000
DcE/dce (R_2r)	D sites: 14 000–16 600
DCe/DCe (R_1R_1)	D sites: 14 500–19 300
DCe/DcE (R_1R_2)	D sites: 23 000–31 000
DcE/DcE (R_2R_2)	D sites: 15 800–33 300
D^ucE/dce (R_2^ur)	D sites: 340–470
D^uCe/D^ucE ($R_1^uR_2^u$)	D sites: 540
D−−/D−−	D sites: 110 000–202 000
cc	c sites: 70 000–85 000
cC	c sites: 37 000–53 000
ee	e sites: 18 200–24 000
eE	e sites: 13 400–14 500

those who are normal Rh D positive. A stronger dosage effect is seen with anti-E and anti-c than anti-D, and the most marked effect is seen in antibodies to compound Rh antigens.

Influence of other Rh antigens

The expression of low frequency antigens often affects the expression of other more common antigens. Low frequency Rh antigens, for example C^w (RH8) and C^x (RH9), will not be discussed here in detail. However, they are usually associated with abnormal expression of one or more of the polymorphic Rh antigens.

In addition, students should be aware of two further effects, commonly known as the cis and the trans effect.

Cis effect

This term is used to describe the observation that when the gene for the D antigen is on the **same** chromosome as a gene for the C or E antigens, the expression of C and E antigens may be depressed. Thus, there is usually more E antigen produced on the red cells of r'' (dcE) than R_2 (DcE) type individuals, and more C antigen on the red cells of r' (dCe) than R_1 (Dce) type individuals.

Trans or Ceppellini effect

This describes the depressed expression of the D antigen due to the presence of the gene for the C antigen on the **opposite** chromosome. For example, red cells from an individual who is type R_1r (DCe/dce) will express more D than red cells of the R_0r' (Dce/dCe) type. In some cases the D antigen may be so depressed as to appear as a D^U.

Weaker forms of Rh antigens

Amino acid substitutions or exon exchanges to produce *RHD/RHCE* hybrid genes can give rise to gene products and conformational changes that result in altered or weakened expression of common antigens. In addition, some individuals express fewer antigens than normal for no apparent reason. Weak expression of the D antigen arises from the expression of a reduced number of D antigen sites on red cells. The D antigen expressed is the same as that expressed by a normal D positive person, that is it carries all the Rh D epitopes, but there is less of it (see Table 5.10). This weakened form of D, historically designated as D^U, is capable of stimulating the production of anti-D in Rh D negative individuals. Failure to detect the weakened D antigen in determining the Rhesus group of blood samples in the transfusion laboratory may result in mistyping blood donors or neonates as Rh D negative. This could result in a Rh D negative patient receiving a transfusion of Rh D positive (D^U) blood or the failure to give anti-D prophylaxis to an Rh D negative mother with an Rh D positive (D^U) infant.

Laboratory aspects of Rh blood group typing

Phenotyping and genotyping

It is often necessary to make an assessment of the phenotype and genotype of an individual when selecting blood for transfusion to patients with Rh antibodies, assessing the likely effect on the foetus of a woman's Rh antibodies or when performing family studies. It is usually possible to derive the genotype from information about the phenotype in Rh D negative individuals. However, with Rh D positive individuals it is usually impossible to tell whether they are homozygous or heterozygous for D and therefore their genotype has to be assumed from the statistically most likely arrangement for their ethnic group. The presence of Rh antigens on red cells is most usually detected using the antisera anti-D, anti-C, anti-E, anti-c and anti-e. The phenotype of an individual may be established from the reactions of their red cells when added to these reagents. Table 5.11

Table 5.11 *Example of the possible genotype of a blood sample using population frequency statistics*

Antisera					Phenotype	Genotype		
-D	-C	-E	-c	-e		*Most likely*	*Less likely*	*Least likely*
+	+	−	+	+	*DCce*	*DCe/dce* R_1r	*DCe/Dce* R_1R_0	*Dce/dCe* R_0r'

+ indicates a positive reaction, − indicates a negative reaction.

Using the example above: The observed phenotype is DCce. The first assumption is that, as no E antigen was detected, then e antigen must be present on both chromosomes. Secondly, as both C and c antigens were detected, they must be located on opposite chromosomes. Thus, the blood sample is phenotypically ?Ce/?ce, where ? = D or **non-D (d)** and '/' divides the two chromosomes. Alternative gene arrangements are:

1. The gene for D is present on both chromosomes and thus the phenotype will be **DCe/Dce** ($R_1R_0 = 2\%$ in Caucasians).
2. The gene for D is present on only one chromosome. This may be either
   (a) the chromosome which carries the gene for C, resulting in the arrangement **DCe/dce**, i.e. type R_1r, found in 33% of Caucasians, or
   (b) the chromosome which carries c, **dCe/Dce**, i.e. type $r'R_0$ which has a frequency of $< 1\%$ in Caucasians.

The most likely genotype is DCe/dce (R_1r), heterozygous with respect to D, though this is not necessarily the correct one. However, it is important to note that if these results were obtained from an individual of the black population, then the genotype DCe/Dce (R_1R_0), homozygous with respect to D, would be the most probable.

The gene arrangement *Dce* (R_0) is much more prevalent in black populations than any other population. In fact it occurs with a frequency of 44% compared to 2% in Caucasians, Orientals and native Americans.

shows an example of the results using Rh antisera and an unknown sample of red cells.

Nature of Rh antibodies

Rh antibodies are usually immune in nature although naturally occurring forms of anti-D, anti-C, anti-E and anti-C^w have been reported. The antibodies may be found in the IgM or IgG form. Anti-D production has even been reported following transfusion of fresh frozen plasma, presumably containing small amounts of red cell membrane. This is due to the high immunogenicity of the D antigen. Antibodies with specificities within the Rh system are often found in cases of autoimmune haemolytic anaemia, e.g. anti-e, anti-C + e, anti-c, anti-c + E.

Anti-D is the most common of all immune blood group antibodies in Rh D negative individuals. It is sometimes found in association with anti-C (anti-C + D) or anti-E (anti-D + E), and rarely with both (anti-C + D + E). In Rh D positive patients, anti-E is often found in R_1r (DCe/dce) and R_1R_1 (DCe/DCe) genotypes. Anti-c and anti-c + E are quite common in R_1R_1 patients. Anti-C and anti-e are much less common.

Antibodies to compound Rh antigens (anti-ce, anti-Ce etc.) may be present in sera containing other Rh antibodies but are difficult to differentiate by routine laboratory tests. Rarely, they may be the sole Rh antibody present in a serum.

Laboratory detection

Immune Rh antibodies often have a wide thermal range. The majority react best at 37°C and are optimally detected using the indirect antiglobulin test or enzyme treated red cells (see Chapter 9). The naturally occurring forms usually react best at lower temperatures. Rh antibodies are not considered to be complement-fixing antibodies.

Clinical significance

Rh antibodies may cause immediate or delayed haemolytic transfusion reactions. In addition, anti-D is still the most common cause of severe HDNB despite anti-D prophylaxis programmes. Anti-c is also recognized as the cause of a significant number of severe cases of HDNB. Rh antibodies are found in many cases of autoimmune haemolytic anaemia. Their deleterious effects cause these antibodies to be of importance in the clinical environment, i.e. they are clinically significant. Antibodies in the Rh system are the most clinically significant of all blood group antibodies apart from the ABO system. The Rh antigens D and c, in particular, are highly immunogenic.

Suggested further reading

Avent, N. (1996). Human erythrocyte antigen expression: its molecular bases. *British Journal of Biomedical Science*, **54**(1), 16–37.

BCSH Blood Transfusion Task Force (1996). Guidelines for pre-transfusion compatibility procedures in blood transfusion laboratories. *Transfusion Medicine*, **6**, 273–283.

Jones, J., Scott, M.M. and Voak, D. (1995). Monoclonal anti-D specificity and Rh D structure: criteria for selection of monoclonal anti-D reagents for routine typing of patients and donors. *Transfusion Medicine*, **5**(3), 171–184.

Sonneborn, H.H. and Voak, D. (1997). A review of 50 years of the Rh blood group system. *Biotest Bulletin*, **5**(4).

Telen, M.J. (1996). Erythrocyte blood group antigens: polymorphisms of functionally important molecules. *Seminars in Haematology*, **33**(4), 302–314.

Yamamoto, F. *et al.* (1990). Molecular genetic basis of the histo-blood group ABO system. *Nature*, **345**, 229–233.

Self-assessment questions

1. List the genes involved in the ABO system and describe their roles.
2. Differentiate between ABH red cell antigens and ABH substances.
3. Compare the frequency of ABO groups in Caucasian, black and Indian populations.
4. Name the genes and their products for the 'two-locus model' of the Rh system.
5. List the five major antigens of the Rh system.
6. What is the thermal range and mode of detection for immune Rh antibodies?

Key Concepts and Facts

- The ABO and Rh systems are the most clinically significant in transfusion science.

- ABO grouping was discovered by Landsteiner and involves antigens on red cells and antibodies in serum to A, B and H.

- ABH antigens are carbohydrate structures attached to the red cell membrane precursor chain by enzymes and production of the enzymes depends on the presence of genes.

- Subgroups of A and B may be detected in certain individuals.

- Secretion of ABH substances depends on the presence of the secretor gene.

- Molecular techniques have given information about the ABO system that has previously been determined from serological techniques.

- The Rh system is controlled by two gene loci: *RHD* (D polypeptide) and *RHCE* (CcEe polypeptide).

- The Rh antigens are expressed as polypeptide chains which span the red cell membrane.

- These polypeptides express numerous epitopes which are important if monoclonal antisera are used for testing, as their specificity may be for a missing epitope – a situation that would lead to a false negative result.

- Rh D antigens are highly immunogenic and immune Rh antibodies may be formed in transfusion incompatibility or in HDNB.

Chapter 6
Other blood group systems

Learning objectives

After studying this chapter you should confidently be able to:

Explain the basis of blood group nomenclature.

List the cellular functions of selected blood group antigens.

Outline the general features of the Lewis, P, Ii, MNSs, Lutheran, Kell, Kidd and Duffy blood group systems.

Describe the clinical and laboratory significance of the blood group antibodies in transfusion, pregnancy and haemolytic disease of the newborn.

List the antigen frequencies in the white and black populations for selected blood groups.

Red blood cells bear numerous cell surface structures that can be recognized as antigens by the immune system of individuals who lack that particular structure. Recipients of a blood transfusion may produce antibodies to an entire structure, or a single or limited number of epitopes. Similarly, a pregnant woman may produce antibodies to foreign antigens expressed on her foetus' red blood cells. More than 600 antigens have been defined on human red cells. The International Society of Blood Transfusion (ISBT) has tabulated 23 blood group systems and five blood group collections. In recent years the biochemical and molecular bases for many of these antigens have been elucidated, as have the biological roles for many blood group antigen structures. In addition, associations between some antigenic phenotypes and disease have been identified. The surface components that are responsible for antigen expression may be divided into carbohydrate and protein structures.

The carbohydrate antigens are expressed by immunodominant sugars which are attached to a precursor molecule by the action of glycosyl transferase enzymes. These enzymes are the products of the blood group genes. The carbohydrate structures are attached covalently to glycolipids or glycoproteins and are synthesized in the Golgi apparatus of erythropoietic cells. The molecular bases of carbohydrate antigens depend on polymorphic variations in the

The key features to be considered for other blood group systems are outlined below.

Antigens
Frequency

General features:

- Whether present at birth.
- Dosage effect.
- Variability of expression.

Disease associations

Antibodies
Nature:

- Immune or naturally occurring.
- Immunoglobulin class.
- Frequency.

Reactions:

- Mode of detection.
- Complement binding.

Clinical significance:

- Transfusion reaction.
- Haemolytic disease of the newborn.

genes that synthesize their glycosyl transferase enzymes, e.g. ABO, Hh, **Lewis, P, Ii.**

Protein antigens are defined by amino acid sequence changes in red cell membrane proteins, which are generated by sequence variation at the DNA level. Broadly they fall into six functional groups:

- Membrane transporters or channels, e.g. Rh, **Kidd**, Diego, Colton, KX.
- Membrane-bound enzymes, e.g. **Kell**, Cartwright.
- Structural or assembly proteins, e.g. **MNSs**, Gerbich.
- Chemokine receptors, e.g. **Duffy**.
- Cell adhesion molecules, e.g. **Lutheran**, LW, Xg, Indian.
- Complement regulatory proteins, e.g. Cromer, Knops, Chido/Rodgers.

The blood group systems covered here are Lewis, P, Ii, Kidd, Kell, Duffy, Lutheran and MNSs (shown in bold type above). At the level of this introductory text, only certain key features for each of these blood group systems will be described.

Blood group nomenclature

Unfortunately, over the years the naming of blood group antigens has been inconsistent and confusing. Originally single letters were used to name blood group antigens such as A and B. The symbol 'O' (standing for zero) meant no antigens were present, until that is, the discovery of H. Single letters continued to be used for the allelic pair M and N, and for P (although now called P_1). This continued with the Rh antigens C, D and E, but with the introduction of lower case letters to describe the allelic pairs of antigens, C and c, D and d, E and e. This system was also used for S and s, K and k, and unfortunately also for I and i which are not an allelic pair. Where subgroups of antigens were identified it became common practice to use subscript numbers, e.g. A_1, A_2, P_1, P_2. The discovery of the Lewis system brought a change to using the first two letters of the propositus' surname (i.e. Le) with the addition of a superscript letter a for the first antigen of an allelic pair to be recognized, and a superscript letter b for the second. Le^a and Le^b, however, were found not to be the products of allelic genes.

This system worked for Duffy and Kidd but, in order to avoid confusion with Rh D, the Duffy antigens were named using the last two letters of the propositus' name (i.e. FY). The Kidd antigens were named using the propositus' initials (i.e. JK) in order to avoid confusion with the K of Kell and Rh D. Similar manipulations of names with superscript letters a, b and most other letters of the alphabet in lower or upper case, continue to be used. In the early 1960s numerical systems were proposed for the antigens of the Kell

Table 6.1 *Some examples of blood group nomenclature*

Blood group system	ISBT No.	ISBT symbol	Gene	Antigen	Antigen positive	Antigen negative	Anti-body
Kidd	009	JK	Jk^a	Jk^a	$Jk(a+)$	$Jk(a-)$	anti-Jk^a
Duffy	008	FY	Fy^a	Fy^a	$Fy(a+)$	$Fy(a-)$	anti-Fy^a
MNSs	002	MNS	M	M	M+	M−	anti-M
P	003	P1	p^{1k}	P_1	P_1+	P_1-	anti-P_1

and Rh systems. Thus phenotypes could be represented by a series of numbers, positive if the antigen was present and negative if the antigen was absent. For example in the Rh system, D = 1, C = 2, E = 3, c = 4, e = 5, so that DCce (R_1r) becomes Rh : 1,2,−3,4,5. These systems carried no genetic implications and proved to be unwieldy in normal conversation.

In 1980 the ISBT set up a Working Party on Terminology for Red Cell Surface Antigens. The aim was to produce a uniform system of terminology which was both eye readable and capable of being adapted for computer use, and in keeping with the genetic basis of the blood groups. Each known antigen was given a unique six digit number, the first three numbers indicating the blood group system and the second three the antigen itself. Existing terminologies were retained and system symbols included. For example, the Kell system is 006 and the K antigen 001, so K may be represented as 006001. Alternatively, the system symbol (KEL) may be used, so that K can also be represented as KEL001. As it is allowable to omit the leading zeros, it is more common to see K represented as KEL1. Table 6.1 shows some examples of blood group nomenclature.

In addition to these variations in naming blood group antigens, there have been problems concerning how the antigens, antibodies and genes should appear on the printed page.

Carbohydrate antigens

Lewis system (ISBT 007, symbol LE)

The antigens Le^a and Le^b are not the products of a pair of allelic genes as the nomenclature might suggest. Indeed they are not true red cell antigens. Lewis antigens are synthesized in secretory tissue (such as gut epithelium) and released into the plasma as soluble glycolipids. They are adsorbed on to the red cell surface from the plasma. The ability to secrete soluble Lewis antigen is independent of the ability to secrete ABH-soluble antigens. ABH secretion is controlled by a separate secretor gene (*Se*) (see Chapter 5). The Lewis gene (*Le*) codes for the production of a transferase enzyme (fucosyl transferase) which attaches fucose to the subterminal

In secretory tissue, the soluble A and B antigen structures may act as substrates for the Lewis transferase, producing the compound antigens ALe^b and BLe^b.

A, B and Lewis transferases all compete for the soluble H antigen structure, so that there is usually less Le^b substance produced and therefore less expressed on red cells in group A, B and AB individuals than in group O individuals.

position of type-1 precursor oligosaccharide. This monofucosylated structure is the Le^a antigen.

In secretory tissue, when the *Se* gene is present, the *H* gene produces a transferase which attaches fucose to the terminal position of type-1 precursor oligosaccharide. This is soluble H antigen. The Lewis transferase then acts by adding a further fucose at the subterminal position of the soluble H antigen. This difucosylated structure is the Le^b antigen.

When the *Se*, *H* and *Le* genes are present, the type-1 precursor has fucose added at the terminal position by H transferase, and at the subterminal position by Lewis transferase, to produce Le^b antigen. In the absence of the *Se* gene, the Lewis transferase adds fucose to the subterminal position to produce Le^a antigen. Thus all Le(b+) individuals are ABH secretors and all Le(a+) individuals are ABH non-secretors.

Individuals who lack any Lewis antigen may be considered to be homozygous for point mutations in the *Le* gene, which results in the production of inactive transferase. Their genotype is usually designated as *lele*. Whether they secrete soluble ABH antigen will depend on whether or not they carry an *Se* gene (see Figure 6.1). Table 6.2 gives a summary of the interactions between *Se*, *Le* and *H* genes.

As described above, Lewis antigens are soluble antigens secreted

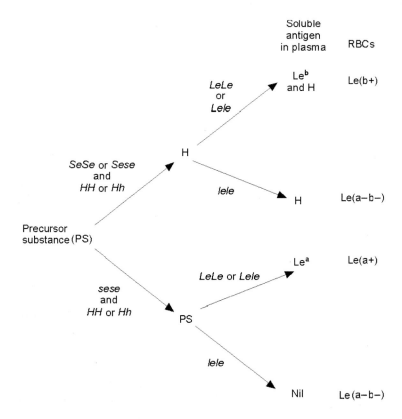

Figure 6.1 *Genetic pathway for Lewis, secretor and H substances in secretory tissue*

Table 6.2 *Summary of interactions between* Se, Le *and* H *genes*

Genotype	Antigens in plasma			Lewis phenotype on RBCs
	ABH	Le^a	Le^b	
SeSe or Sese LeLe or Lele HH or Hh	+	+ small amount	+	Le(a−b+)
sese LeLe or Lele HH or Hh	−	+	−	Le(a+)
SeSe or Sese LeLe or Lele hh	−	+	−	Le(a+)
sese LeLe or Lele hh	−	+	−	Le(a+)
SeSe or Sese lele Hh or Hh	+	−	−	Le(a−b−)
sese lele HH or Hh	−	−	−	Le(a−b−)
SeSe or Sese lele hh	−	−	−	Le(a−b−)
sese lele hh	−	−	−	Le(a−b−)

into plasma and reversibly adsorbed on to red cells. This means that Lewis antigen can be lost from red cells when blood samples are stored. When testing cells for Lewis antigen or sera for Lewis antibodies, it is therefore advisable to use the freshest available red cells. Similarly, because the Lewis antigen is found in plasma and the supernatant suspending medium of stored red cells, cells must be washed in saline prior to testing to avoid the soluble antigen neutralizing Lewis antibody in the test or typing serum.

Lewis system antigens

General features

The Lewis antigens are produced in secretory tissue. They also appear as soluble antigens in plasma and are reversibly adsorbed on to red cells. The Lewis antigens may weaken or disappear during pregnancy and this is thought to be due to the change in the lipoprotein composition of blood. Sometimes Lewis antibodies are also detected in the plasma. However, these antibodies

Table 6.3 *Population frequency of Lewis system antigens*

	Frequency (%)	
	Whites	*Blacks*
Le(a+b−)	22	23
Le(a−b+)	72	55
Le(a−b−)	6	22

disappear when the normal Lewis phenotype is restored after the birth of the infant.

The **Le^a** antigen, discovered in 1946, shows variable expression from individual to individual and is unstable on storage. Le^a antigen is not detected on newborn red cells but as they mature from a few weeks to 6 months, 80–90% of infants appear Le(a+). They begin to express their true Lewis type with increasing age. The Lea substance may be taken up from plasma on to Le(a−) red cells making them appear Le(a+).

The **Le^b** antigen, discovered in 1948, is weak or absent at birth and is not well detected on red cells until 3 years of age, and it is also unstable on storage. The Le^b substance may be taken up from plasma on to Le(b−) cells. Le^b antigens are more easily detected on red cells from blood groups O and A$_2$ than on those from blood group B, although they are more difficult to detect on red cells from blood groups A$_1$ and A$_1$B. This is due to competition from A and B transferases for the H antigen. Table 6.3 indicates the frequency of Lewis antigens in the population and Table 6.4 illustrates the features of Lewis antibodies.

Disease associations

The Le^b antigen acts as a receptor for the micro-organism *Helicobacter pylori* which has been isolated from the stomach of some patients who suffer from gastritis and appears to cause peptic ulcers and cancer. The mucosal surface of the stomach contains receptors to which *H. pylori* binds. These receptors contain fucose, which is in fact the Le^b and H antigen.

P system (ISBT 003, symbol P1) and Globoside Collection (ISBT 209, symbol GLOB)

Discovered in 1927 by Landsteiner and Levine during animal experiments, the P antigen system has proved to be more complex than the Lewis system.

As with all the carbohydrate antigens, the sugars which express the different antigens in the P system are attached to a precursor oligosaccharide by the action of glycosyl transferase enzymes. So far

Table 6.4 *Clinical and laboratory features of Lewis system antibodies*

	Anti-Le^a	Anti-Le^b
Immune or naturally occurring	Naturally occurring in Le(a−b−) individuals	Naturally occurring in Le(a−b−) and rarely in Le(a+b−) individuals
Immunoglobulin type	Usually IgM	IgM
Frequency	Common antibody	Common antibody
Detection	Well detected with enzyme tests	Well detected with enzyme tests
	Usually a cold agglutinin, but may be a 37°C agglutinin	Usually a cold agglutinin, but may be a 37°C agglutinin
Complement binding	May bind complement	Some examples bind complement
	May cause *in vitro* haemolysis of Le(a+) cells	
Haemolytic transfusion reaction (HTR)	May cause HTR	Unlikely to cause HTR
Haemolytic disease of the newborn (HDNB)	Does not cause HDNB	Does not cause HDNB
General	Usually of low titre	Classically show stringy agglutination of red cells
	Classically show stringy agglutination of red cells	

the molecular bases underlying these transferases are unknown. The antigens to consider are P_1, P and P^k.

P_1 is now considered as the only true antigen of the P system, the antigens P and P^k having been assigned to the Globoside Collection by the ISBT. The P^k antigen is produced by the action of a transferase which adds galactose to a ceramide dihexose (CDH) precursor, converting it to a ceramide trihexose (CTH). The P antigen is produced by the action of a transferase which adds *N*-acetylgalactosamine to CTH, converting it to a globoside (see Figure 6.2). The addition of these P sugars makes the P^k antigen less accessible to its antibody, which may explain why P^k is difficult to detect on P+ red cells in the laboratory. The P_1 antigen is produced by the action of a transferase which adds galactose to a paragloboside precursor. This precursor is closely related to both CDH and the precursor oligosaccharide chain of the ABH antigens.

Table 6.5 *Genes and gene products of the P system, based on the Graham and Williams two-locus model*

Gene	Allele	Gene product	Action
Locus 1	p^k	α-Galactosyl transferase	Converts CDH to CTH (P^k)
	p^{1k}	α-Galactosyl transferase	Converts CDH to CTH (P^k)
			Converts paragloboside to P_1
	p	None	None
Locus 2	p^2	β-Galactosyl transferase	Converts CTH (P^k) to globoside (P)
	p^{20}	None	None

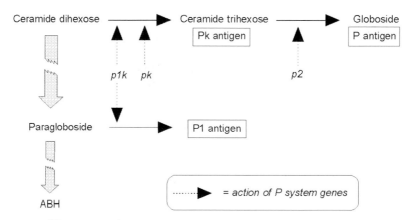

Figure 6.2 *Development of P system antigens*

Figure 6.2 shows the development of the P system antigens. The genes and gene products of the P system are described in Table 6.5, Table 6.6 shows the P system antibodies and Table 6.7 lists the P system phenotypes, antigens and antibodies.

P system antigens

General features

The frequency of the P_1 antigen in white populations is 79% and in black populations is 93%. The P_1 antigen shows variable

Table 6.6 *Clinical and laboratory features of P system antibodies*

	Anti-P_1	*Anti-P*	*Anti-PP_1P^k (Tjᵃ)*
Immune or naturally occurring	Naturally occurring	Naturally occurring	Naturally occurring
Immunoglobulin type	IgM	IgM	IgM
Frequency	Common in P_1 individuals	Found in rare P^k+ individuals	Found in rare pp individuals
Detection	Cold agglutinin Well detected in enzymes	Wide thermal range Well detected using enzyme tests	Wide thermal range Well detected using enzyme tests
Complement binding	A few examples bind complement at 37°C	Most bind complement at 37°C Some are haemolytic at 37°C	Most bind complement at 37°C and cause haemolysis
Haemolytic transfusion reaction (HTR)	May cause HTR if complement bound at 37°C	May cause HTR if complement bound at 37°C	May cause HTR
Haemolytic disease of the newborn (HDNB)	Does not cause HDNB	Does not cause HDNB	Does not cause HDNB
General	**Autoanti-P** may be found as the biphasic IgG associated with paroxysmal cold haemoglobinuria. It binds to red cells in the cold and causes haemolysis when warmed to 37°C		

Table 6.7 *P system phenotypes, antigens and antibodies*

Phenotype	Antigens	Possible antibodies	Frequency (%)
P_1	P_1 and P	–	Whites 79
			Blacks 93
P_2	P	anti-P_1	Whites 21
			Blacks 7
p	–	anti-PP_1P^k	Rare
P_1^k	P_1 and P^k	anti-P	Very rare
P_2^k	P^k	anti-P, anti-P_1	Most rare

expression from weak to very strong in different individuals. The P_1 antigen is not fully expressed at birth. Both P_1 and P^k substance have been found in the fluid derived from a hydatid cyst, a cyst that develops from infection by the migratory tapeworm *Echinococcus granulosus*. P_1 substance has been found in red cells, plasma and droppings from pigeons and in the white of turtle doves' eggs.

Disease associations

P system antigens have been found on urinary tract epithelium where they may act as receptors for micro-organisms such as *Escherichia coli* and so play a role in the pathogenesis of some cases of urinary tract infection and pyelonephritis. In addition, the P antigen is the cellular receptor for the B19 parvovirus, a virus which does not usually cause disease but may be transmitted in blood and in rare cases inhibits red cell production.

Ii system (ISBT 207, symbol Ii)

Discovered in 1956 by Wiener and associates, I and i are not antithetical antigens but common related structures. They are both high frequency antigens whose expressions are inversely proportional to one another. Foetal and neonatal red cells express the i antigen with little detectable I antigen. During the first 18 months of life, the expression of i slowly decreases and that of I increases.

The I and i antigens are defined by a series of carbohydrates on the inner portion of ABH oligosaccharide type-2 precursor chains. I is expressed by the branched structure and i by the linear structure. The i antigen is synthesized by the action of β-3-*N*-acetylglucosaminyl transferase and β-4-*N*-acetylgalactosyl transferase on the paragloboside-derived precursor chain. The i antigen is converted to the I structure by the branching enzyme β-6-*N*-acetylglucosaminyl transferase. As branched chains form, anti-i no longer has good access to its antigen and therefore i antigen expression appears to decrease as I antigen develops.

Most adults express large amounts of I antigen and have very little expression of i antigen. Rarely, adults continue to express i antigen rather than I antigen. This may be due to the inability to produce the branching enzyme, a recessive trait. Two types of adult i phenotype have been described:

- i_1, which has the least amount of i antigen expression and is associated with Whites.
- i_2, which has a little more i antigen expression and is associated with Blacks.

The I and i antigens are widely distributed throughout the body, having been found on lymphocytes, granulocytes, monocytes and platelets as well as on red cells. The antigens have also been found in saliva, milk, plasma, amniotic fluid, urine and ovarian cyst fluid. Thus, normal adults are positive for the I antigen (I+) and neonates are positive for the i antigen (i+).

The clinical and laboratory features of the antibodies in the Ii system are shown in Table 6.8. For further discussion of the role of Ii antibodies in autoimmune haemolytic disease, see Chapter 7.

Compound carbohydrate antigens

The biochemical structures that define ABH, Lewis, P and Ii antigens are very similar. It is therefore not surprising that many antibodies have been described which react with compound antigens from these carbohydrate antigen systems. Examples of these compound antigens are ALe^b, BLe^b, IA, IB, IH, iH, IP_1, iP_1 and ILe^{bH}. The antibodies to these compound antigens require both antigens to be present for the antibody to react.

Protein antigens

MNSs system (ISBT 002, symbol MNSs)

There are 38 antigens in this system, four of which will be considered in this chapter: M, N, S and s. The antigens M and N were discovered in 1927 during experiments which involved injecting human red cells into rabbits to elicit an immune response. The S antigen was discovered in 1947 and the s antigen in 1951. These antigens were detected in human blood using the indirect antiglobulin technique (IAT). The antigens M, N, S and s are produced by two codominant allelic pairs of genes *MN* and *Ss* occurring at two closely linked loci. The gene combinations *MS*, *Ms*, *NS* and *Ns* are inherited intact and can be traced through families. *MS* is more common than *Ms* and *Ns* is more common than *NS*.

The M and N antigens are expressed on red cell glycophorin A (GPA) and the S and s antigens on glycophorin B (GPB). The antigens differ due to amino acid substitutions on the N-terminal

Table 6.8　*Clinical and laboratory features of the antibodies in the Ii system*

	Autoanti-I	Autoanti-i
Immune or naturally occurring	Naturally occurring	May be found secondary to infections such as infectious mononucleosis, or diseases involving the reticulo-endothelial system
Immunoglobulin type	IgM	IgM (rarely IgG)
Frequency	Present in all normal sera	See above
Detection	Enhanced in enzyme tests	Enhanced in enzyme tests
	Cold agglutinin	Cold agglutinin
	May be ABO group specific	Identified by titration against adult and cord red cells, Anti-i will react with both adult and cord red cells, but to a much higher titre with cord red cells
	Identified by titration against adult and cord red cells. Anti-I will react with both adult and cord red cells, but to a much higher titre with adult red cells	
Complement binding	May bind complement and cause haemolysis *in vitro*	May bind complement
Haemolytic transfusion reaction (HTR)	May cause HTR	
Haemolytic disease of the newborn (HDNB)	Does not cause HDNB	May cause mild HDNB
General	Most common autoantibody found in cold haemagglutinin disease. May be very high titre with extended thermal range	
	May be found with raised titre secondary to infection, especially with *Mycoplasma pneumoniae*	
	Alloanti-I is a naturally occurring cold agglutinin in the very rare adult I individuals	

portion of GPA and GPB. The glycophorins are sialoglycoproteins which contribute greatly to the net negative charge of the red cell membrane. This negative charge prevents red cells from adhering to one another or to vessel walls. It seems possible that GPA acts as an assembly point for the biosynthesis of red cell membrane proteins such as band 3 protein and that GPB plays a similar role in the assembly of the Rh complex.

MNSs system antigens

The population frequency of the MNSs system antigens is shown in Table 6.9.

General features

The MNSs antigens are well developed on the red cells at birth. They show a marked dosage effect when present in the

Table 6.9 *Population frequency of the MNSs antigens*

	Frequency (%)	
	Whites	*Blacks*
M+N−	28	26
M+N+	50	44
M−N+	22	30
M−N−	Rare	Rare
S+s−	11	3
S+s+	44	28
S−s+	45	69
S−s−	0	<1

Table 6.10 *Clinical and laboratory characteristics of MN system antibodies*

	Anti-M	*Anti-N*
Immune or naturally occurring	Naturally occurring	Naturally occurring
Immunoglobulin type	IgM and IgG	IgM and IgG
Frequency	Fairly common	Very rare
Detection	Usually cold agglutinin	Usually cold agglutinin
	May act in IAT at 37°C	May act in IAT at 37°C
	Not detectable with enzymes	Not detectable with enzymes
	Reactions often enhanced at pH below 6.5	
Complement binding	Unlikely to bind complement	Unlikely to bind complement
Haemolytic transfusion reaction	May cause HTR if reactive at 37°C	May cause HTR if reactive at 37°C
Haemolytic disease of the newborn	May cause mild HDNB	May cause HDNB

homozygous state. The antigens of the MNSs system are destroyed by treatment with enzymes in the laboratory (see Chapter 9).

The clinical and laboratory features of the MNSs antibodies are summarized in Tables 6.10 and 6.11.

Disease associations

Glycophorin A (MN) acts as a receptor for the malarial parasite *Plasmodium falciparum*. Red cells lacking GPA have long been noted to resist invasion by *P. falciparum*.

Table 6.11 *Clinical and laboratory characteristics of Ss system antibodies*

	Anti-S	Anti-s
Immune or naturally occurring	Immune	Immune
Immunoglobulin type	IgG and IgM	IgG
Frequency	Uncommon antibody	Uncommon antibody
Detection	May act as a cold agglutinin	Best detected in IAT at 37°C
	Best detected in IAT at 37°C	Variable reactions with enzymes
	Variable reactions with enzymes	
Complement binding	May bind complement	May bind complement
Haemolytic transfusion reaction (HTR)	May cause HTR	May cause HTR
Haemolytic disease of the newborn (HDNB)	May cause mild to severe HDNB	May cause mild to severe HDNB

Lutheran system (ISBT 005, symbol LU)

There are 20 antigens in or associated with the Lutheran system. Only two, Lu^a discovered in 1946 and Lu^b discovered in 1956, will be described in this text. The Lutheran antigens are expressed on red cell membrane glycoprotein structures which probably play a role in cell adhesion during erythropoiesis. The codominant allelic genes *Lu^a* and *Lu^b* are closely linked to the secretor gene locus on chromosome 19. This linkage was the first example of autosomal gene linkage in humans to be described. The minus–minus phenotype, Lu(a–b–), in which neither Lu^a nor Lu^b antigen is expressed on the red cell, may occur by one of three mechanisms:

- By the inheritance of an unlinked, dominant inhibitor gene *In(Lu)*.
- By the inheritance of a silent (*lu*) gene from both parents.
- By the inheritance of a recessive, sex-linked inhibitor gene *XS2*.

The Lutheran system antigens show variable expression from individual to individual. They are poorly developed at birth and are not very immunogenic. The population frequency for the Lutheran system is shown in Table 6.12. The clinical and laboratory features of antibodies to the Lutheran system are summarized in Table 6.13.

Kell system (ISBT 006, symbol KEL)

The Kell system antigens are expressed on a red cell membrane glycoprotein which has membrane-bound enzyme activity. There are 24 antigens in or associated with the Kell system of which six

Table 6.12   *Population frequency of the Lutheran system antigens*

| | Frequency (%) | |
	Whites	Blacks
Lu(a+b−)	0.15	0.1
Lu(a+b+)	7.5	5.2
Lu(a−b+)	92.35	94.7
Lu(a−b+)	Rare	Rare

will be considered. They result from the codominant, allelic pairs *K* and *k*, *Kp^b* and *Kp^b*, *Js^a* and *Js^b*. These three pairs of alleles are closely linked.

The antigen K, originally called Kell, was discovered in 1946. It was named after Mrs Kellacher who developed an antibody in her serum which reacted with the red cells of her husband, her elder daughter and her newborn infant. In 1949, k, also known as Cellano, was discovered, followed by Kp^a, also known as Penney, in 1957. Two further antigens in the system, Kp^b, also known as Rautenberg, and Js^a, also known as Sutter, were discovered in 1958. The antigen Js^b, also known as Matthews, was discovered in 1963.

Kp^a is associated with Caucasian and Js^a with black populations.

Individuals who phenotypically express both K and Kp^a antigens always carry the corresponding *K* and *Kp^a* genes on different chromosomes. The presence of the Kp^a antigen has been shown to suppress the expression of k and Js^b antigens.

There is a rare, silent, recessive gene, K_0, which produces no Kell antigens. Individuals who are of the K_0K_0 genotype express no Kell antigens and, if immunized by exposure to a Kell antigen, may produce an antibody known as anti-K_U. It is not certain whether

Table 6.13   *Clinical and laboratory characteristics of Lutheran system antibodies*

	Anti-Lu^a	*Anti-Lu^b*
Immune or naturally occurring	Naturally occurring or immune	Immune
Immunoglobulin type	IgM and IgG	IgM and IgG
Frequency	Not very common	Rare
Detection	May act as cold agglutinins	May act as cold agglutinins
	May act in IAT at 37°C	Most act in IAT at 37°C
	Variable reactions with enzymes	Variable reactions with enzymes
Complement binding	May bind complement	May bind complement
Haemolytic transfusion reaction (HTR)	Unlikely to cause HTR	May cause HTR
Haemolytic disease of the newborn (HDNB)	May cause mild HDNB	May cause mild HDNB
General	Mixed field agglutination	Mixed field agglutination

Table 6.14   *Population frequency of the Kell system antigens*

	Frequency (%)	
	Whites	*Blacks*
K+k−	0.2	<0.1
K+k+	8.8	3.5
K−k+	81	96.5
Kp(a+b−)	<0.1	<0.1
Kp(a+b+)	2	<0.1
Kp(a−b+)	98	>99
Js(a+b−)	0.1	1
Js(a+b+)	0.1	18
Js(a−b+)	>99	81

this antibody reacts with a 'total' or 'universal' Kell antigen, or is a mixture of many Kell antibodies. The presence of the K_0 gene on one chromosome depresses the expression of Kp^a by the opposite chromosome (trans effect). There is also a sex-linked gene, *XK*, which encodes the antigen K_X. Although K_X is not a Kell system antigen, its presence is required for the normal expression of Kell antigens.

Table 6.14 shows the population frequency of the antigens in the Kell system. The clinical and laboratory characteristics of the antibodies are summarized in Table 6.15.

In conclusion, the general features of this system are that K is the most immunogenic antigen outside the ABO and Rh systems, Kell system antigens are well developed at birth and Kell system antigens show some dosage effect but this is not very marked or consistent.

Duffy system (ISBT 008, symbol FY)

The Duffy blood group antigens are expressed on a red cell membrane glycoprotein with chemokine receptor activity. Of the six antigens in the Duffy system, only those resulting from the codominant, allelic pair Fy^a and Fy^b will be considered. The Fy^a antigen was discovered in 1950, and Fy^b in 1951. The minus–minus phenotype, Fy(a−b−), occurs in individuals homozygous for the silent gene *Fy*. This phenotype is very rare in Whites but occurs in 68% of Blacks of African descent. The Duffy antigens are interesting in that they are the site of attachment to the red cell for the malarial parasites *Plasmodium vivax* and *Plasmodium knowlesi*. Thus the Fy(a−b−) genotype is an advantage to those living in areas where malaria is endemic.

Duffy system antigens

The population frequency of the Duffy system antigens is shown in

Table 6.15   *Clinical and laboratory characteristics of Kell system antibodies*

	Anti-K	*Anti-k (Cellano)*
Immune or naturally occurring	Immune	Immune
Immunoglobulin type	IgM and IgG	IgM and IgG
Frequency	Common in transfused patients	Rare
Detection	Variable results in enzymes	Variable results in enzymes
	May act as a cold agglutinin	Best detected in IAT at 37°C
	Usually best detected in IAT at 37°C	
Complement binding	May bind complement	May bind complement
Haemolytic transfusion reaction (HTR)	Causes HTR	Causes HTR
Haemolytic disease of the newborn (HDNB)	Causes HDNB	Causes HDNB

	Anti-Kp^a (Penney)	*Anti-Kp^b (Rautenberg)*
Immune or naturally occurring	Immune	Immune
Immunoglobulin type	IgG	IgG
Frequency	Rare	Very rare
Detection	Variable results in enzyme tests	Variable results in enzyme tests
	Best detected in IAT at 37°C	Best detected in IAT at 37°C
Complement binding	May bind complement	May bind complement
Haemolytic transfusion reaction (HTR)	Causes HTR	Causes HTR
Haemolytic disease of the newborn (HDNB)	Causes HDNB	Causes HDNB

	Anti-Js^a (Sutter)	*Anti-Js^b (Matthews)*
Immune or naturally occurring	Immune	Immune
Immunoglobulin type	IgG	IgG
Frequency	Rare	Very rare
Detection	Variable results in enzyme tests	Variable results in enzyme tests
	Best detected in IAT at 37°C	Best detected in IAT at 37°C
Complement binding	May bind complement	May bind complement
Haemolytic transfusion reaction (HTR)	Causes HTR	Causes HTR
Haemolytic disease of the newborn (HDNB)	Causes HDNB	Causes HDNB

Table 6.16. The antigens are well developed at birth and are moderately immunogenic. The clinical and laboratory features of antibodies in the Duffy system are summarized in Table 6.17. It should be noted that, in laboratory tests, the antibodies are destroyed using enzyme techniques (see Chapter 9).

Disease associations

Duffy antigens form the site of attachment for the malarial parasite *Plasmodium vivax* to red cells.

Table 6.16   *Population frequency of the Duffy system antigens*

	Frequency (%)	
	Whites	*Blacks*
Fy(a+b−)	17	9
Fy(a+b+)	49	1
Fy(a−b+)	34	22
Fy(a−b−)	0	68

Table 6.17   *Clinical and laboratory characteristics of the Duffy system antibodies*

	Anti-Fy^a	*Anti-Fy^b*
Immune or naturally occurring	Immune	Immune
Immunoglobulin type	IgG	IgG
Frequency	Not uncommon in transfused patients	Rare
Detection	Not detectable using enzyme techniques	Not detectable using enzyme techniques
	Best detected in IAT at 37°C	Best detected in IAT at 37°C
Complement binding	May bind complement	May bind complement
Haemolytic transfusion reaction (HTR)	May cause HTR	May cause HTR
Haemolytic disease of the newborn (HDNB)	May cause HDNB	May cause HDNB

Kidd system (ISBT 009, symbol JK)

The Kidd blood group antigens are expressed on a red cell membrane glycoprotein which has urea transport activity across the red cell membrane. There are three antigens in the Kidd system, of which only those resulting from the codominant, allelic pair Jk^a and Jk^b, will be described here. The Jk^a antigen was discovered in 1951, and Jk^b in 1953.

The minus–minus phenotype, Jk(a−b−), occurs in individuals who are homozygous for the silent gene *Jk*. This phenotype is rare in both black and white populations (see Table 6.18). In laboratory tests, a marked dosage effect can be demonstrated. The Kidd

Table 6.18   *Population frequency of the Kidd system antigens*

	Frequency (%)	
	Whites	*Blacks*
Jk(a+b−)	27	57
Jk(a+b+)	50	34
Jk(a−b+)	23	9
Jk(a−b−)	Rare	Rare

Table 6.19 *Clinical and laboratory characteristics of the Kidd system antibodies*

	Anti-Jk^a	Anti-Jk^b
Immune or naturally occurring	Immune	Immune
Immunoglobulin type	IgM and IgG	IgM and IgG
Frequency	Not uncommon in transfused patients	Less common than anti-Jk^a
Detection	Enhanced in enzyme tests Best detected in IAT at 37°C	Enhanced in enzyme tests Best detected in IAT at 37°C
Complement binding	Bind complement	Bind complement
Haemolytic transfusion reaction (HTR)	May cause HTR Common antibody in cases of delayed HTR	May cause HTR
Haemolytic disease of the newborn HDNB	May cause mild HDNB	May cause mild HDNB
General	Unstable on storage of blood samples Antibody levels in patients often fall very quickly	Unstable on storage of blood samples Antibody levels in patients often fall very quickly

antigens are well developed in the newborn and can be detected on their red cells. The antibodies of the Kidd system are described in Table 6.19.

Importance of other blood groups in transfusion science

It is necessary for the transfusion scientist to be aware of the importance of the blood groups described in this chapter. The detection of antibodies in transfused patients who have been given ABO- and Rh-compatible blood products is usually due to the transfusion of red cells containing antigens from one of the above blood group systems. Tests must then be performed to identify the antibodies and knowledge of the antibody characteristics is required. An awareness of the clinical significance of the antibody is important in issuing compatible blood for transfusion in order to prevent unwanted reactions (see Chapter 10). Consideration of the frequency of the antigen in the population is also necessary, for example in selecting suitable blood for transfusion that lacks a particular antigen. There are many important aspects for discussion relating to blood groups systems. This chapter has examined some of them at an introductory level.

Suggested further reading

Avent, N.D. (1996). Human erythrocyte antigen expression: its molecular bases. *British Journal of Biomedical Science*, 54(1), 16–37.

BCSH Blood Transfusion Task Force (1996). Guidelines for pre-transfusion compatibility procedures in blood transfusion laboratories. *Transfusion Medicine*, **6**, 273–283.

Daniels, G. (1995). *Human Blood Groups*. Oxford: Blackwell Scientific Press.

Harmening, D.M. (1996). *Modern Blood Banking and Transfusion Practices*. Philadelphia: F.A. Davis Company.

Moulds, J.M., Nowicki, S., Moulds, J.J. and Nowicki, B.J. (1996). Human blood groups: incidental receptors for viruses and bacteria. *Transfusion*, **36**, 362–374.

Telen, M.J. (1996). Erythrocyte blood group antigens: polymorphisms of functionally important molecules. *Seminars in Haematology*, **33**(4), 302–314.

Self-assessment questions

1. Which blood group antigens are carbohydrate structures?
2. Which blood group antigens are protein structures?
3. Describe how the I and i antigens differ.
4. List the antibodies that are able to bind complement to red cells.
5. Which blood groups have a connection with malaria?

Key Concepts and Facts

- Blood group antigens may be carbohydrates or proteins.

- Specific roles within the red cell membrane have been identified for most of the blood group antigens.

- Antibodies will be produced by an individual when they are exposed to a foreign blood group antigen.

- It is important to be aware of the clinical significance of antibodies to blood group antigens, particularly those which are haemolytic, bind complement or act at body temperature.

- The population frequencies of blood group antigens are of significance when selecting blood products or blood components for transfusion.

Chapter 7

Immune/autoimmune haemolytic anaemia and haemolytic disease of the newborn

Learning objectives

After studying this chapter you should confidently be able to:

Describe the effects of antibody attachment on red blood cells.

Define immune and autoimmune haemolytic anaemia.

Define three mechanisms of immune haemolytic anaemia due to drugs.

Discuss the underlying mechanisms of the disorders.

Discuss the historical developments in haemolytic disease of the newborn (HDNB).

Describe the role of the maternal response in how the disorder occurs.

Describe how the disorder affects the foetus or newborn infant.

Outline the methods used to establish the presence of immune disorders.

Outline the strategies for HDNB prophylaxis.

A brief explanation of the mechanisms of red cell destruction is needed to understand the importance of inappropriate red cell antibody production and the clinical significance to patients. Normal red cell breakdown occurs in the liver and spleen (extravascular) when the cells become aged or damaged. The haemoglobin is further degraded into its components haem and globin. The molecules of haem are converted to bilirubin which is dealt with by the liver. Thus the possibility of free haemoglobin or its products in the circulating blood is avoided. When this occurs intravascularly there are mechanisms for binding and removing the haem or haemoglobin in order to prevent subsequent damage to the kidneys. Raised blood levels of breakdown products, such as bilirubin, haem or haemoglobin, suggest haemolysis of red cells due to a pathological defect. These may be estimated by the laboratory to investigate a possible haemolytic episode. A raised bilirubin level is evident in a patient as the yellow skin colour of jaundice.

Immune and autoimmune red cell antibodies may attach to the corresponding antigenic component on the red cell membrane, sometimes involving the fixation of complement components as well. This results in inappropriate red cell breakdown which may be intravascular or extravascular. As red cell destruction is increased, the bone marrow responds by increasing the release of immature red cells into the circulation. This is demonstrated in the peripheral blood film by the presence of nucleated red cells, reticulocytes and/ or polychromasia, all of which indicate the presence of immature red cells. When the bone marrow no longer has the capacity to compensate, anaemia develops in the patient as shown by a lowered red cell count and haemoglobin level. The increase in haemolysis is detectable by increased plasma bilirubin levels (extravascular) and the presence of free plasma haemoglobin (haemoglobinaemia) with haemoglobin in the urine (haemoglobinuria) in severe cases.

Causes and classification of the immune haemolytic anaemias

The immune haemolytic anaemias (IHAs) may occur as a result of production of an antibody in response to a foreign stimulus, for example a blood transfusion that is incompatible or drug treatment. These types are called immune haemolytic anaemias. Auto-immune haemolytic anaemias also may occur, usually by the production of antibodies stimulated by disease processes, or the presence of malignant cells or substances produced during a disease. They are called **primary** or **idiopathic** disorders if no apparent cause for their existence can be identified and **secondary** if the cause is known. Those IHAs which are drug induced have a special category and will be described in more detail later.

The autoimmune haemolytic anaemias are classified into two types according to the temperature at which the antibodies react optimally with red cells. This is called the **thermal range. Warm-type** AIHA antibody combines with the red cells at any temperature but most rapidly at 37°C. **Cold-type** AIHA antibody combines optimally at 0–20°C and shows a decreased affinity to attach to the red cells as the temperature increases.

The laboratory detection of antibodies bound to red cells *in vivo* can be demonstrated by the direct antiglobulin test (DAT) which is described in Chapter 9.

The incidence of warm AIHA varies. Primary cases, which are not the result of another disorder, account for 48% of all cases, whereas drug-induced IHAs account for approximately 8%. Secondary causes include lymphomas and disorders such as systemic lupus erythematosus (SLE), rheumatoid arthritis, pernicious anaemia, hepatitis and colitis, plus some miscellaneous causes. The incidence in females is greater than in males. Some of the known disease associations for the warm and cold types are further described below.

Warm antibody types

- AIHA in children: This is usually an acute disease following viral infection. Most patients recover, though a few develop a condition which persists, usually associated with deficiencies of immunoglobulin such as IgA.

- AIHA with thrombocytopenia: An IgG type antibody develops which is specific for platelet antigens.

- AIHA and tumours: The relationship between the tumour and autoantibody production is unclear. However, removal of the tumour seems to cure the disorder. Tumours of the ovaries and thymus may cause AIHA, though this is rare.

- AIHA secondary to diseases: Systemic lupus erythematosus (SLE) sufferers may develop a red cell autoantibody and 10% show a positive DAT. The antibody type is IgG and complement fixing, and occasionally it shows Rh specificity. Hodgkin's disease and lymphoma patients may produce an autoantibody which is also capable of fixing complement to the red cells, and thus a few cases are DAT positive. Similarly, a small number of patients with chronic lymphocytic leukaemia are DAT positive as they have produced an IgG antibody which is probably of the Rh type.

Cold antibody types

Chronic cold haemagglutinin disease accounts for approximately 45% of cold antibody type immune disorders. Infectious mononucleosis (glandular fever) is caused by the Epstein–Barr virus and accounts for about 30%; other disorders such as lymphoma and paroxysmal cold haemoglobinuria (PCH) are also implicated.

Chronic cold haemagglutinin disease

The antibody that is present in these patients is an IgM which is specific to the I antigen found on all adult red cells. It always activates complement and is thus very haemolytic. Antibody binding occurs when the patient's skin temperature drops below 28–30°C. Haemoglobinuria, haemosiderinuria, haemoglobinaemia and jaundice occur as a result of intravascular haemolysis. However, the haemolysis of red cells only occurs when the peripheral circulation (such as fingertips and toes) is restored to body temperature, as the blood becomes warm. The antibody dissociates from the red cells at 37°C but the activated complement components are still attached. If haemolysis does not occur immediately then the complement-coated red cells will be removed by the **reticuloendothelial system** (see Chapter 1).

> An antibody is described as high titre when the serum containing the antibody is diluted, usually by a series of doubling dilutions in saline, and shows agglutination at dilutions greater than 1 in 64, with red cells expressing the corresponding antigen.

Cold autoantibodies and infection

The presence of cold autoantibodies may be due to infection, particularly with *Mycoplasma pneumoniae*. This causes an acute haemolytic anaemia due to the anti-I antibody which has a high thermal range. In infectious mononucleosis only a few cases develop haemolysis and this is related to **high titre** anti-i autoantibodies reacting at cold temperatures. Adult red cells exhibit the 'I' antigen (see Chapter 6) and are not usually affected by anti-i. Why a small number of patients develop haemolysis is not clear.

Paroxysmal cold haemoglobinuria (PCH)

This is a rare condition in which the thermal range of the antibody is 15–17°C. This means that there must be considerable chilling before haemolysis of the red cells begins. The antibody is known as the Donath–Landsteiner antibody (after the workers who first described it in 1904) and it activates complement. Acute anaemia develops rapidly as haemoglobin is freed from red cells undergoing haemolysis in the blood vessels and is lost in the urine (haemoglobinuria). This is one of the consequences of intravascular haemolysis. A secondary condition may occur, usually associated with viral infection, in which there is one attack of haemolysis and the antibody titre falls within a week. The antibody in PCH appears to be anti-P and is of the IgG class. It has a biphasic action in that it attaches to red cells at cold temperatures, such as that in cold fingers and toes, but red cell breakdown occurs as complement is fixed to the cell membrane at normal body temperature. It is extremely haemolytic to the patient's red cells.

Causes of immune/autoimmune haemolytic anaemias

There are a number of possible mechanisms that could contribute to the antibody production in these patients, as outlined below.

- **Genetic factors.** The incidence in families is low, but some cases do occur and thus it is likely that a genetic predisposition to develop AIHA may exist.
- **Modified red cell antigens.** It is possible that viruses, bacteria or some metabolite could enter the red cell membrane or expose hidden antigens, so giving rise to antibodies reactive with the red cell surface.
- **Cross-reacting antibodies.** These are antibodies associated with infection that may also cause AIHA. The autoantibody in these cases is short-lived and is polyclonal, suggesting a response to an infection.
- **Failure to recognize and eliminate autoreactive clones.** Many different antibody specificities are generated by a mutation of the somatic (body) cells during early life. This results in a series of lymphocytes which can form distinct antigen-recognition units on their cell surface and these recognition units can compete for specific antigens. It is thought that autoreactive lymphocytes that are capable of proliferating into clones of plasma cells producing autoantibody are eliminated or paralysed during the establishment of tolerance. It seems that self-antigens can normally interact with the autoreactive lymphocytes as they arise, a process which may be part of the body's essential defence against disease. Autoantibodies may arise as a result of the proliferation of clones of small lymphocytes to which tolerance could not be established or maintained.

Drug-induced haemolytic anaemia

The drug-induced haemolytic anaemias may be divided into two main types. The first type induce the formation of antibodies directed against the drug (or metabolite), or some drug–protein complex. These are known as the immune haemolytic anaemias and the antibody can be detected only if the drug is present The second type induce the formation of antibodies against antigens on the red cell membrane and the presence of the drug is not required for antibodies to be detected. This type produces a haemolytic anaemia that is caused by an autoimmune antibody.

Immune haemolytic anaemia (IHA)

Drugs are low molecular weight substances and are not likely to induce antibodies directly. However, they are transported in the body by a firm chemical coupling of the drug to a protein carrier. The protein that acts as the carrier may or may not be a component of the tissue which is damaged by the resulting anti-drug antibody formed. Two methods are described to explain the mechanisms by which the drugs induce antibody formation.

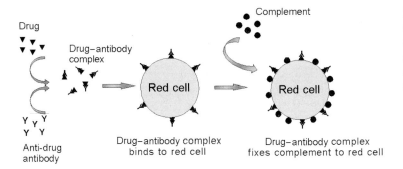

Figure 7.1 *The immune complex mechanism. Anti-drug antibodies form a complex with the drug which then binds to the red cell membrane. This causes complement to be bound to the red cell and leads to haemolysis*

Immune complex mechanism

This is also called the **innocent bystander mechanism**. Most of the drugs that induce antibodies act by this method. Common examples are quinine, quinidine, *p*-aminosalicylic acid and phenacetin. An antibody is produced which then combines with the drug, and the drug–antibody complex attaches to the cell surface. This induces the binding of complement to the red cells and so haemolysis occurs (see Figure 7.1). Thus the protein carrier allows the drug to act as a hapten. It has been suggested that either the drug is bound to the cell membrane of the target cell, or that a drug–plasma protein complex is formed. It seems that IgM antibodies are associated with the destruction of red cells and IgG antibodies with platelet destruction as far as quinidine is concerned. Platelets have Fcγ receptors but red cells do not. However, red cells have C3b receptors which facilitate the uptake of complement.

Only a small quantity of drug will result in rapid intravascular haemolysis in a sensitive person. It appears that these immune complexes bind reversibly to the target cells and can migrate from cell to cell, fixing complement at each stop. This would explain the massive effect of small amounts of drug. The antibody is usually IgM, though it can be IgG, and binds complement.

Drug adsorption (hapten) mechanism

This mechanism differs in that drugs such as penicillin and cephalothin are strongly bound to the red cell membrane and are present on the cells of all patients taking large doses of the drug. This coating is not damaging in itself, but some patients develop high titre antibodies which attack the cell-bound penicillin and result in haemolysis. The major hapten (see Chapter 2) in penicillin is the benzylpenicilloyl (BPO) group and over 90% of normal patients have anti-BPO antibodies. In most cases these antibodies are IgM but those associated with haemolytic anaemia are IgG. Large doses of penicillin and cephalothin are required for antibodies to be produced, and the haemolysis develops more slowly and is not intravascular. The antibody is usually of the IgG class

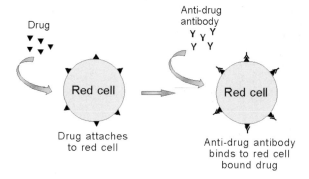

Figure 7.2 *The drug adsorption mechanism. The drug attaches directly to the red cell membrane by adsorption. Antibodies to the drug are produced and bind to the red cell bound drug*

and complement is not involved. Figure 7.2 illustrates the basis of the drug adsorption mechanism.

Membrane modification or non-immunologic protein adsorption involves the non-specific adsorption of plasma proteins onto the membrane of red cells which have been sensitized by a drug, for example cephalothin. These proteins include IgG, IgM and IgA, and the acute phase proteins α_1-antitrypsin, α_2-macroglobulin, fibrinogen and complement components C3 and C4. This adsorption may not lead to haemolytic anaemia but it can confuse the results when a patient is investigated as the DAT becomes positive. This mechanism is shown in Figure 7.3.

Cephalothin is unique among drugs in that it can cause a positive DAT by three different mechanisms. As well as the mechanism previously described, anti-cephalothin antibodies may be produced as described for penicillin, or cephalothin-coated red cells may cross-react with anti-penicillin antibodies.

Autoimmune haemolytic anaemia

AIHA associated with methyldopa occurs in approximately 20% of patients treated for raised blood pressure with the drug methyldopa (Aldomet). Patients develop a positive DAT due to the formation of an auto IgG antibody. A small number develop haemolytic anaemia. The DAT may continue to be positive up to 18 months

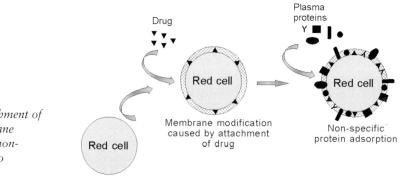

Figure 7.3 *The membrane modification mechanism. Attachment of the drug to the red cell membrane modifies it in such a way that non-specific plasma proteins are also adsorbed*

after stopping the drug treatment. The antibody often shows Rh specificity, usually anti-c or anti-e.

Laboratory tests for diagnosis of autoimmune/immune haemolytic anaemia

In order to diagnose AIHA it is necessary to show the following in the laboratory:

- That the antibody present in the patient's serum sample has been bound *in vivo* to the patient's red cells. This would be shown by a positive DAT. In addition, after eluting the antibody, i.e. removing it from the red cells, it has a specificity which makes it capable of agglutinating red cells of other individuals with the same phenotype.
- That the patient's red cells have a shortened lifespan. This indicates that active haemolysis is occurring.
- that the antibodies are present in the patient's serum and are similar to those on the patient's red cells.

Sometimes not all of these criteria may be met, for example:

- Cold antibodies may only be detectable by their ability to activate complement.
- The autoantibody may not show any specificity.
- The antibody may be reacting with a drug.
- A positive DAT may be found without anaemia if the patient has been able to compensate for the haemolysis by a response in the bone marrow to increase red cell production.

Haemolytic disease of the newborn (HDNB)

Many years ago it was not uncommon for an infant to be stillborn. One of the common causes for the failure of these infants to survive was described in 1939 by Philip Levine and Rufus Stetson. They described the passage of antibodies from the mother to the foetus and the syndrome was later defined as 'rhesus haemolytic disease of the newborn'. Prior to treatment, 1 in 200 pregnant mothers developed Rh antibodies and a fifth of these lost their infants in the first pregnancy, with the rate increasing dramatically in subsequent pregnancies to leave just over half of the infants surviving.

Haemolytic disease of the newborn (and of the foetus) is caused by production of an antibody in the mother in response to an antigen carried on the red blood cells of the developing baby. If some trauma occurs during the pregnancy and the baby's red cells cross into the mother's circulation it is known as a **transplacental haemorrhage** (TPH) or a **foetal-maternal haemorrhage** (FMH). This

> Philip Levine and Rufus Stetson published a paper in the *Journal of the American Medical Association* called 'An unusual case of intra-group agglutination'. It was reprinted some 40 years later in *Vox Sanguinis* (1980) and hailed as a milestone in the history of medical science.

Figure 7.4 *Haemolytic disease of the newborn in an Rh D positive foetus and Rh D negative mother. Foetal red cells that are Rh D positive enter the maternal circulation. Anti-D is produced by an immune response in the Rh D negative mother. The IgG anti-D crosses the placenta into the foetal circulation and attaches to the foetal red cells causing haemolysis*

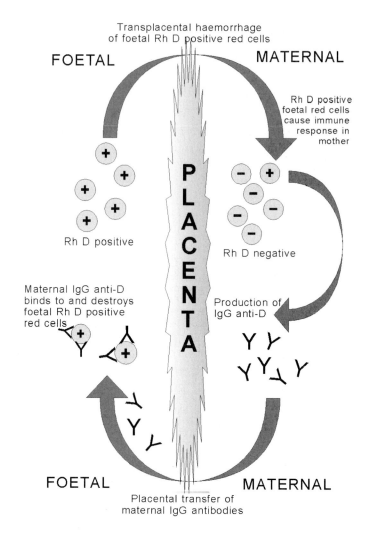

can also occur as a normal consequence of birth. The placental barrier excludes antibodies of the IgM class but will allow IgG antibodies to cross due to the presence of Fc receptors on the cell membrane of the placental cells to which the antibodies bind. The antibody produced by the mother is transported across the placenta into the foetal circulation. The antibody then attaches to the foetal red cells and causes haemolysis to occur in the foetal circulation. This can result in haemolytic disease of the newborn, depending upon a number of factors. The strength of the antibody that is developing in the maternal circulation must be regularly checked so that steps can be taken to prevent or minimize the effects of the antibody in the foetal blood. An illustration of how HDNB occurs is shown in Figure 7.4.

The clinical effects of haemolysis on the baby

The attachment of IgG antibodies to the foetal red cells results in their agglutination and destruction by the reticuloendothelial system which in the foetus involves macrophages in the foetal circulation or spleen. They phagocytose the antibody-coated and agglutinated red cells. The foetus or neonate suffers from the events that occur during intravascular haemolysis. The haemoglobin levels fall due to decreased red cell survival and serum bilirubin levels are raised. These are regularly measured by the laboratory. Bilirubin is a breakdown product of haemoglobin so this is an indication of how much haemolysis is taking place in the baby's circulation. If the levels of unconjugated bilirubin become too high the result will be brain damage due to **kernicterus**. In this situation, the baby may be placed under a source of ultraviolet light to speed up the breakdown of bilirubin. Normal levels of unconjugated bilirubin are less than $17\,\mu\mathrm{mol}\,l^{-1}$, although in normal newborn infants the level may reach $85\,\mu\mathrm{mol}\,l^{-1}$. Levels of $350\,\mu\mathrm{mol}\,l^{-1}$ or more are not uncommon and are highly toxic to the brain. The levels of bilirubin are more of a problem after the baby is born because prenatally it is cleared via the placenta. The neonatal liver is not sufficiently mature to conjugate the bilirubin and render it non-toxic. In this instance, it may be necessary to exchange the total blood volume of the baby with fresh donor blood. An exchange transfusion has a number of beneficial effects and is straightforward to perform.

If the baby is severely affected prior to birth the result is intrauterine death from **hydrops foetalis**. Hydrops foetalis is a condition that causes stillbirth. The foetus is very pale and swollen with fluid in the body cavity and brain which results in mental damage and death. In its moderate form the disease results in the baby being born with severe anaemia and jaundice. Mildly affected babies show a slight anaemia and possibly some jaundice.

> Kernicterus comes from the words 'kernel' and 'icterus'. Kernel, meaning nucleus in German, refers to the brain and icterus (Latin) refers to the yellow pigment, in this case due to bilirubin. Bilirubin has an affinity for the lipids present in the brain tissue and therefore causes damage, particularly in babies.

Test to detect antibodies formed by the mother

Although haemolytic disease of the newborn can be caused by a number of IgG antibodies, the most frequently described antibody involved in the disease is the Rh antibody, anti-D. This is an IgG antibody and is therefore likely to cause foetal damage if produced. Mothers who are Rh D negative lack the D antigen on their red cells. However, if the father is Rh D positive, the D antigen may be inherited by the baby. A father who is homozygous, i.e. of genotype **DD**, can only pass the gene for the D antigen to the baby, which will then be heterozygous for the D antigen, with the genotype Dd. However, if the father is Rh D positive but heterozygous, the baby is equally likely to inherit the genotype **dd**. So it is important first to identify the genotype of the father to see if there is a likelihood that the baby is carrying the D antigen. The mother is then checked regularly throughout her pregnancy for the production and level of

Chorionic villus sampling is a technique that involves taking a sample from the placenta and can be performed from the eighth week of pregnancy. It is performed via a catheter inserted through either the cervix or the abdomen during ultrasound examination. Other techniques for assessing the foetus are foetal blood sampling using cordiocentesis, and amniocentesis to estimate levels of antibodies in the amniotic fluid.

antibodies. If the titre of antibodies rises to a dangerous level in her circulation then clearly the foetus is at risk. As a rough guide, anti-D levels greater than $5 \, \text{i.u.} \, \text{ml}^{-1}$ are indicative of risk. However, it is important to note that a number of factors are involved, such as the mother's previous obstetric history, how fast the development of antibodies has occurred and the type or subclass of IgG involved. Tests on the foetus include **amniocentesis** where some amniotic fluid is withdrawn from the foetal sac through a needle inserted into the abdominal wall of the mother. The bilirubin pigment in the fluid may be measured using a spectrophotometer. This gives an estimation of the amount of red cell destruction taking place. The Rhesus status of the foetus can be identified using the technique of **chorionic villus sampling** during the first 3 months of pregnancy to obtain a sample of foetal cells, which are then tested using methods such as **flow cytometry, solid phase microfluorescence** or the **polymerase chain reaction** for the presence or absence of the D antigen or other antigens that may be foreign to the mother.

Exchange transfusion

As stated earlier, it may be necessary to replace the baby's blood with fresh blood. This may be performed as a prenatal or postnatal procedure. The donor blood selected for exchange transfusion must be less than 5 days old and have a haematocrit of approximately 0.5–0.6 (see Chapter 8). The blood should be irradiated to inactivate the donor lymphocytes in order to minimize the risk of transfusion-related graft versus host disease in the foetus or neonate. Blood for transfusion is checked for compatibility by cross-matching with the maternal serum. The technique is performed by removing small volumes of the neonatal or foetal blood and simultaneously infusing donor blood. The beneficial effects of exchange transfusion are as follows: circulating antibodies and sensitized red cells are diluted or removed, the haemoglobin level is raised to a normal value, and the bilirubin levels are lowered thus preventing further risk of damage. The British Committee for Standards in Haematology has produced guidelines for the transfusion of neonates.

Prophylactic disease prevention

Prophylaxis (i.e. prevention) stops a disease occurring before the events that cause it have happened. The prophylaxis of Rh haemolytic disease of the newborn has been a great success story. At the start of the 1960s a meeting took place in Liverpool, UK, during which it was suggested that the destruction of foetal cells in the mother's blood might be possible by injecting an antibody into the mother after the birth of the baby.

Rhesus prophylaxis with anti-D has dramatically reduced the

number of deaths due to haemolytic disease of the newborn, and the number of registered deaths for this disorder in England and Wales fell from 106 in 1977 to 11 in 1990. A standard dose of 500 International Units (IU) of immunoglobulin is routinely given to all Rh negative mothers who have carried or delivered a Rh D positive infant. This is sufficient to destroy the red cells resulting from an FMH of less than 4 ml of foetal blood. Larger doses are required if the FMH has been greater. The way in which the volume of foetal blood is estimated is described later. In order to be effective it is important that prophylactic anti-D is given to mothers of all Rh positive babies within 72 hours of giving birth and to all Rh negative pregnant women following amniocentesis, chorionic villus sampling, miscarriage, induced abortion, ectopic pregnancy or any trauma to the abdomen. Each of these events is likely to cause FMH. The mechanism of action of prophylactic anti-D is that it attaches to the foetal Rh D positive circulating cells in the mother which are then trapped in the spleen.

Quantitation of foetal-maternal haemorrhage

There are a variety of methods available to determine whether FMH has occurred and to estimate the amount of foetal red cells in maternal blood.

The standard formula used to determine the volume of FMH is based on the number of foetal cells multiplied by the maternal blood volume and divided by the number of maternal cells. To estimate the number of foetal cells the most popular test is still the Kleihauer–Betke stain which was first described in 1957. This is a simple technique based on the principle that the haemoglobin in foetal cells is resistant to elution from the red cells when placed in an acid environment. On the other hand, the haemoglobin contained in adult red cells is removed by the action of an acid pH. In the Kleihauer–Betke stain, a smear of maternal blood is placed in a solution of haematoxylin and hydrochloric acid to lower the pH to about 1.5, and then counterstained with eosin. The result is that the maternal red cells appear as 'ghosts', with only the red cell stroma remaining, while foetal cells stain a deep pink and leukocytes stain blue/grey. The ratio of foetal to maternal red cells is counted under a microscope and the extent of foetal haemorrhage can be calculated. Other methods for determining the number of foetal cells include flow cytometry and immunofluorescence. These techniques are usually more time consuming and expensive but highly accurate.

Other antibodies and haemolytic disease of the newborn

The most common cause of HDNB is incompatibility of the ABO blood group system between mother and infant, although this

Professor Sir Cyril Clarke was famous for his work at Liverpool University on the mechanics of Rhesus sensitization in red cells. His workers had noted a correlation between the incidence of sensitization by Rhesus antibodies in maternal blood samples and the number of foetal red cells in the mother's circulation. The Rhesus negative mothers became sensitized by a small amount of foreign (foetal) Rhesus positive blood during their pregnancy. It had also been noted that Rh sensitization was much reduced when there was incompatibility of the ABO group between mother and baby, for example, a group O mother and group A father, resulting in a group A baby. It was reasoned that the naturally occurring anti-A (or anti-B) destroyed the foetal cells as soon as they entered the mother's circulation. Thus the mother was less likely to become sensitized to Rh D positive cells. Therefore to introduce anti-D into the mother's blood would have the same effect as the anti-A or anti-B, that is, to destroy Rh D positive cells. In a clinical trial, the expected result was found, i.e. the mother did not become sensitized and her immune system was not stimulated to produce anti-D.

A group of American workers published similar findings using a passive anti-D to prevent active immunization on exposure to the antigen. They too found that this procedure had a protective effect.

scenario is not as clinically significant as Rh HDNB. If the mother produces IgG anti-A or anti-B in response to the baby's A, B or AB red cells, then these antibodies are able to cross the placenta and damage the foetal cells. The clinical effect of HDNB due to ABO antibodies is less pronounced, and usually a raised bilirubin level may be seen 1–3 days after birth. ABO incompatibility can occur in the first pregnancy and any further pregnancies. Haemolysis can also occur due to the action of other IgG antibodies and occasionally anti-C, anti-c, anti-E, anti-e, anti-K or anti-Fy^a may be implicated, as well as various other irregular antibodies. There are approximately four deaths per year in the UK from HDNB caused by anti-c or anti-K. HDNB due to anti-K has a slightly different mechanism in that the anaemia is caused by suppressed red cell production rather than haemolysis.

The success of anti-D immunoprophylactic treatment has meant that there are more occurrences of mild or moderate HDNB due to non-RhD antibodies. Sometimes the symptoms do not develop in these infants until a few days after birth, so it is important to screen for antibodies in pregnant women who may be at risk.

Suggested Further Reading

Harmening, D.M. and Prihoda, L.E. (1994). Autoimmune haemolytic anaemias. In *Modern Blood Banking and Transfusion Practices* (ed. D.M. Harmening). Philadelphia: F. A. Davis Company.

Kennedy, M.S. (1994). Hemolytic disease of the newborn and fetus. In *Modern Blood Banking and Transfusion Practices* (ed. D.M. Harmening). Philadelphia: F. A. Davis Company.

Tovey, I.A.D. (1996). Haemolytic disease of the newborn and its prevention. In *ABC of Transfusion* (ed. M. Contreras). London: BMJ Publishing Group.

Self-assessment questions

1. Define warm haemolytic anaemia and give examples of diseases in which it may occur.
2. List the likely causes of cold haemolytic anaemia.
3. Describe the process of red cell haemolysis.
4. Differentiate between the mechanisms of drug-induced haemolytic anaemia.
5. Describe the effects of kernicterus and how it may be prevented.
6. List the situations where prophylactic anti-D immunoglobulin should be given to a mother.
7. Explain the principle of the Kleihauer–Betke test.

Key Concepts and Facts

- Autoimmune/immune haemolytic anaemias are caused by the production of either warm- or cold-reacting antibodies by the patient.

- This results in the breakdown of red cells, known as haemolysis, and thus anaemia develops.

- Antibody production may be stimulated by diseases, infections, drugs or foreign red cells as in HDNB.

- Drug-related immune/autoimmune haemolysis occurs via three mechanisms: the immune complex or innocent bystander mechanism, drug adsorption, and the induction of red cell autoantibodies.

- HDNB is caused by maternal antibodies produced in response to foetal red cells presenting an antigen that stimulates the maternal immune system.

- The antibodies produced are type IgG and transfer across the placenta to damage the foetal red cells.

- This causes haemolysis and results in the symptoms of HDNB such as anaemia and hyperbilirubinaemia.

- Prophylactic treatment has been highly effective in the case of Rh D negative women with Rh D positive infants.

Chapter 8
Blood products and components

Learning objectives

After studying this chapter you should confidently be able to:

List the components derived from blood.

Describe the physiological role of each component.

Discuss the processing and use of components and products derived from plasma.

Describe the storage of blood products.

Discuss the importance of quality control procedures.

Colloid osmotic activity is largely provided in the blood by the physiological concentration of albumin, which accounts for 60–80% of the normal colloid osmotic pressure of plasma. The dynamics between circulating blood and extracellular fluid levels in the tissues were described by Starling in 1896. His work showed that the plasma proteins had oncotic activity, i.e. colloid solutions were able to remain in the blood vessels rather diffuse into the tissues. This is of particular importance when the capillaries and tissues are damaged such as in a burns patient. By transfusing a colloid solution such as albumin the circulating volume can be maintained and transport can occur effectively. A state known as haemorrhagic shock results if the circulating volume is insufficient, i.e. the patient is hypovolaemic. Tissues become **ischaemic** (starved of oxygen) and tissue damage, or **necrosis**, occurs.

The most effective way to make optimum use of a unit of blood is to separate it into its various components. The patient can then be transfused with the component in which they are deficient. This strategy results in a wider availability of blood products and components and has the advantage that the patient is exposed to fewer transfusion-related risks. This chapter will discuss the products available, their production process and clinical use, and the procedures developed to prevent blood-transmitted infections.

The basic physiological role of blood is to provide volume for circulation and the transport of many substances and cellular elements. By cellular elements we mean the blood cells – red cells (erythrocytes), white cells (leukocytes) and platelets (thrombocytes). The volume is made up by plasma, which contains proteins such as fibrinogen, albumin and globulin (including the immunoglobulins). These large molecules provide the plasma with **colloid osmotic pressure.**

In addition the plasma contains the coagulation factors. From a transfusion aspect these are the essential components that may be transfused to a patient in need. Table 8.1 lists the products and components available from whole blood for transfusion to a patient. The clinical requirements of a patient are important in deciding which blood product is transfused. A patient who has

Table 8.1 *Products and components available from whole blood for transfusion*

Components available from whole blood	Products derived from pooled plasma
Red cell concentrates*	Human albumin solution
Platelet concentrates	Immunoglobulins
Fresh frozen plasma	Coagulation factor concentrates
Cryoprecipitate	Prothrombin complex concentrate

* Includes red cells in CPDA1, SAG-M red cells, SAG-M buffy coat depleted red cells and leuko-depleted red cells.

sustained a **massive blood loss,** for example following surgical or obstetric haemorrhage or a road traffic accident, has two major requirements: to replace the lost volume and to provide oxygen carrying capacity. Blood volume may be replaced by a number of fluids, e.g. human albumin solution, saline, colloid solutions or whole blood. Oxygen carrying capacity is provided by red blood cells, so the patient may be given whole blood or a red cell concentrate. There are few clinical reasons for whole blood to be the component of choice; most units of donor blood are separated into components. Massive blood loss would also need replacement of coagulation factors that have been lost during haemorrhage. Fresh frozen plasma contains high levels of coagulation factors and will be described later in this chapter.

Other clinical situations that can involve transfusion are pre- and post-surgical procedures. Prior to a surgical operation, the patient's haemoglobin level, red cell count and **haematocrit** are measured by the laboratory to ensure that these parameters are normal, as there will be further blood loss during surgery.

A 'top up' of red cell concentrate (also known as packed red cells) may be needed. Similar parameters are checked post-surgery and further transfusion of red cells may be required, as well as coagulation factors either in the form of fresh frozen plasma or as specific clotting factors.

There are many haematological examples in which a patient may suffer from **anaemia** without haemorrhage. These include dietary deficiencies, such as of iron, vitamin B12 or folic acid, or genetic disorders involving ineffective haemoglobin synthesis, for example thalassaemia. Disorders affecting the bone marrow, such as leukaemia and aplastic anaemia, result in ineffective haemopoiesis and leukopoiesis. Furthermore, the treatment for these disorders can prevent normal bone marrow activity, resulting in anaemia or a low platelet count. In such cases much support therapy is required involving blood products, especially red cells, platelets and coagulation factors.

The haematocrit (Hct) is a ratio obtained by measuring the volume of plasma and the volume of packed red blood cells after the unit or patient sample of blood has been centrifuged. It is sometimes called the packed cell volume, or PCV. The mean value for males is 0.47 and for females 0.42 (expressed as a ratio per litre of plasma to litre of red cells). It is much higher in neonates due to the increased haemoglobin levels at birth. A unit of donated blood may have the haematocrit checked to ensure it is adequate for transfusion to a patient.

A solution of citrate, phosphate and dextrose is used to prevent the donor blood from clotting. Adenine is also added to maintain ATP levels. Citrate is commonly used for its anticoagulant properties as it removes calcium ions, which are required for the coagulation factors to form a clot.

The additive solution SAG-M is commonly used in the UK. It consists of: sodium chloride at $140\,mmol\,l^{-1}$ – a diluent of physiological concentration, and adenine ($1.5\,mmol\,l^{-1}$), glucose ($50\,mmol\,l^{-1}$) and mannitol ($30\,mmol\,l^{-1}$) – to maintain the ATP levels required for red cell metabolism and prevent haemolysis of red cells.

The use of SAG-M allows virtually all of the plasma to be removed. This means that more plasma can be made available for fractionation into products. The Hct of SAG-M red cells ranges between 0.50 and 0.70. However, as most of the plasma proteins have been removed the viscosity is reduced.

Red cell concentrates

Red cell concentrates are obtained from individual units of donor blood by centrifugation and removal of the plasma. The volume of plasma removed will determine the haematocrit of the product. If the haematocrit is high then the blood is more viscous and may cause problems in transfusion, particularly to neonates or the elderly. Red cells contain the oxygen carrying molecule haemoglobin (Hb). The balance between the portion of oxygen circulating bound to Hb and the portion released to the tissues is regulated by 2,3-diphosphoglycerate (2,3-DPG), which is present in nearly equimolar amounts in the red cells. It acts by lowering the affinity of Hb for oxygen at the concentration normally present in red cells. Thus oxygen is released to the tissues as blood circulates in the capillary bed. The anticoagulant into which the donor blood is taken must ensure that sufficient quantities of 2,3-DPG are maintained for the length of time that the blood will be held for transfusion. A solution of **citrate, phosphate and dextrose-adenine (CPDA1)** is normally used for anticoagulation and preservation.

The expiry period for red cell concentrates is 35 days if stored at $4°C$. As the blood ages, the 2,3-DPG levels, and therefore the oxygen carrying capacity, are reduced. A combination of preservative substances may be added to the red cells to prolong metabolic activity and levels of 2,3-DPG. This is called an 'additive solution' and consists of saline, adenine containing glucose and mannitol, and is known as **SAG-M**. Red cells with SAG-M added are less viscous and therefore easier and quicker to transfuse.

A rise of approximately $10\,g\,l^{-1}$ of haemoglobin should be seen in the patient for each transfused unit of red cells.

Leukocyte-depleted blood components

Leukocytes transmit viruses, express HLA antigens and produce cytokines. For these reasons they may cause infection (particularly with cytomegalovirus), non-haemolytic febrile transfusion reactions and alloimmunization to HLA. Some patients are susceptible and may have already been exposed to antigens of the HLA system, or are immunosuppressed due to their illness or treatment, or perhaps are requiring or recovering from a stem cell transplant. A strong indication for the depletion of leukocytes in blood components is to prevent the recurrence of **non-haemolytic febrile transfusion reactions** (see Chapter 10) in certain patients, and to prevent alloimmunization to HLA.

Leukocytes are removed from the blood by filtering through a leukocyte-specific filter prior to transfusion. This may occur at either the blood centre, the hospital blood transfusion laboratory, or the bedside as the transfusion is given. The aim is to remove sufficient leukocytes from the red cell or platelet donation to prevent adverse effects, and a residual level of less than 5×10^6 leukocytes per unit of red cells (or adult therapeutic dose of platelets) is considered to be satisfactory. Leukocyte-depleted products may be used as an alternative to cytomegalovirus (CMV) negative products in cases where the viral transmission of CMV is to be avoided for patients at risk. Transfusion of infants below 1 year of age and neonates should always be with leukocyte-depleted blood components. This also applies to intrauterine transfusions.

The uncertainty surrounding the transmission of prion-related disease, i.e. new variant Creutzfeldt–Jakob disease, has further implicated the white cells as possible carriers. Thus it is likely that all blood and blood products will be leuko-depleted by filtration procedures soon after donation has taken place. These issues are rapidly changing and the student is advised to be aware of the importance of constantly updating current practices to meet the needs that arise from environmental issues in society.

Washed red cells

A unit of red cells will also contain some residual plasma, as well as the leukocytes and platelets discussed above. Plasma proteins are present, such as IgA, which may react in a patient who has previously formed anti-IgA. Other examples are patients who are found to have allergic reactions to transfusion for no apparent reason or have developed autoimmune haemolytic anaemia. In this case antibodies are causing haemolysis which is enhanced by the presence of complement. These are very rare clinical disorders in which adverse reactions to transfusion may be avoided by washing the donated red cells in saline. Thus all traces of plasma proteins are removed.

Plasma-derived blood components

The separation of blood into the cellular components and plasma by centrifugation has been explained earlier. This will also occur if the blood is left to sediment naturally although the process takes much longer. The speed of centrifugation determines whether cellular components will be present in plasma as the cells sediment according to their differences in density, size and ability to deform. This means that if the blood is centrifuged at a high relative centrifugal force (RCF) the red cells, leukocytes and platelets will eventually be forced to the lower portion, leaving a virtually cell-free plasma component. Plasma has the lowest density with a specific gravity of $1026\,\mathrm{g\,cm^{-3}}$ when compared with water at $20°C$, but red cells have a specific gravity of $1100\,\mathrm{g\,cm^{-3}}$. The majority of leukocytes, which are less dense than red cells, sediment at the interface between the red cells below and the plasma above.

Figure 8.1 *A unit of blood after centrifugation, showing the relative volumes of each component*

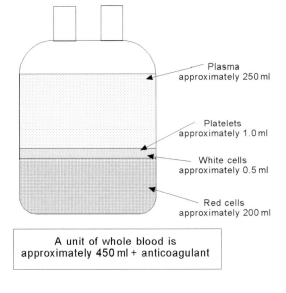

Plasma
approximately 250 ml

Platelets
approximately 1.0 ml

White cells
approximately 0.5 ml

Red cells
approximately 200 ml

A unit of whole blood is
approximately 450 ml + anticoagulant

This is known as the 'buffy layer'. Careful removal of the plasma, without disturbing this layer, should result in a leukocyte- and platelet-depleted volume of plasma, known as platelet-poor plasma (PPP). Platelets are the smallest and least dense of the blood cells and therefore take the longest to sediment. If blood is centrifuged at a lower RCF the platelets remain in the upper layer of plasma. This results in a plasma component which is 'platelet-rich' (PRP), to be discussed later in this chapter.

In blood transfusion practice the aspiration of plasma components is performed in a 'closed system' to prevent infection of the blood by exposure to the environment. The plastic containers into which the blood is taken from the donor vein are specially made with a series of 'ports' to which plastic tubing has been attached so that a number of components can be removed from the original donor unit using an aseptic technique (see Figure 8.1).

Plasma fractionation

The technique of separating plasma into its components was first described by Cohn in 1944. Plasma (platelet-poor) may be pooled from large numbers of donors or used as an individual product. Pooled plasma is used to obtain a variety of components for treating patients. Currently, approximately 450 tonnes of plasma are sent to the Bio-Products Laboratory each year from England and Wales.

Human albumin solution

The role of albumin in the body is primarily to provide colloid osmotic activity and to act as a binding protein for various substances including bilirubin, lipids, metallic ions and drugs.

Cohn was working at the Harvard Protein Laboratory when he developed a protein purification system which was initially used with bovine plasma. Extensive supplies of plasma had been required during the Second World War and albumin was thought to be the plasma protein that was most effective in providing oncotic activity. The protein purification technique was based on solid/liquid separation techniques using cold ethanol fractionation. He used a reaction medium in which the conditions, such as temperature, hydrogen ion concentration and ionic strength, were carefully controlled. Cold ethanol was added to partition the main proteins by their presence either in the precipitate or supernatant. This technique, further modified, has long been used on a large scale in the Bio-Products Laboratory at Hertfordshire, UK, to provide plasma proteins.

Low levels of albumin result from the shock and trauma associated with blood loss or severe burns. Albumin was first used in the Second World War to treat the many casualties as an alternative to whole blood. Albumin is produced from cold ethanol fractionation using pooled plasma donations at the Bio-Products Laboratory in the UK. It is filtered and heated to 60°C for 10 hours so that any viruses present are inactivated. It is then stored for 2 weeks at 30–32°C and examined for bacterial contamination. It is a safe, though expensive, plasma component with a shelf-life of 2–3 years when stored between 2 and 25°C.

Immunoglobulins

Immunoglobulins are obtained either from blood donation or by the process of plasmapheresis. Donors are tested for the presence of immunoglobulins, particularly high titres of IgG antibodies, in their blood. The specific immunoglobulin can then be injected into patients with immunoglobulin deficiency or used as a prophylactic for a number of infectious diseases including tetanus, hepatitis B and cytomegalovirus. It can be stored for up to 12 months at 4–6°C. Prophylactic anti-D immunoglobulin, as given to Rh D negative mothers, is also provided. However, there is increasing interest in antibody-producing recombinant cell lines for supplying immunoglobulins.

Coagulation factor concentrates

It is necessary to understand the process of **haemostasis,** which literally means 'to stop bleeding', so that the importance of providing coagulation factor concentrates can be appreciated. Clotting factor VIII is formed in the hepatocytes of the liver and has a role in the coagulation cascade. When converted to its activated form it allows the process to continue until fibrin is formed. In this way haemorrhage is prevented. A simplified scheme of blood coagulation is shown in Figure 8.2.

Clinical indications for the transfusion of factor VIII are haemophilia A, von Willebrand's disease and acquired deficiency of factor VIII. Each of these disorders and the transfusion requirements will be described in more detail. Haemophilia A is a congenital deficiency of factor VIII which may be mild, moderate or severe. It results in haemorrhage, particularly into the joints, and is very painful. The factor VIII gene is found on the X chromosome and mainly affects males, though females may be carriers or, rarely, sufferers of the disorder. Gene mutations include premature stop codons and deletions within the 26 exons. The most severe defect occurs as a result of a mutation pattern in intron 22 in which DNA transcription is disrupted so that no functional factor VIII is formed. A similar haemorrhagic disorder, von Willebrand's

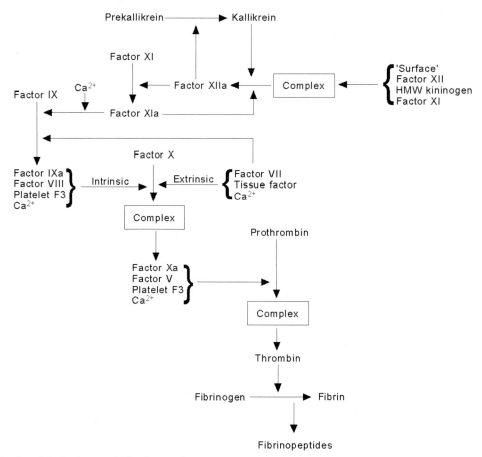

Figure 8.2 *Simplified scheme of blood coagulation*

disease (vWd), has an autosomal dominant inheritance pattern. The defect results in the inability to form von Willebrand factor (vWf), a cofactor to which factor VIII must be bound in the circulation. Without the presence of vWf the clotting cascade cannot proceed to fibrin formation. The treatment for these disorders is to infuse factor VIII concentrate, so restoring this factor in the blood to levels which are effective in haemostasis. One of the problems of factor VIII infusion is that approximately 20% of haemophiliacs develop inhibitory antibodies to human factor VIII concentrate. However, other sources of factor VIII are available such as animal, especially porcine, or recombinant factor VIII.

The process of plasma-derived factor VIII production in the UK takes place at the Bio-Products Laboratory where the plasma is pooled from donors. Approximately 6 tonnes of plasma are used for each batch. It is essential to inactivate or remove viruses in plasma, especially when large donor pools are involved and the risk of virus transmission is increased. Inactivation is achieved during the fractionation process itself and also by heating to 80°C for 72 hours or by chemical treatment.

Recombinant factor VIII is produced from cell lines, for example hamster ovary or kidney cells, which are grown in a culture medium. The cells have had the human gene for factor VIII inserted so that factor VIII is produced and can then be harvested, purified (using chromatography) and heated or chemically treated to inactivate viruses.

Ultimately it is likely that treatment will be available in the form of gene therapy for these disorders.

Other factor concentrates

Whilst most of the clotting factors are available through both plasma fractionation and recombinant DNA technology, factor VII and factor IX concentrates (which include factors X and II, protein C and protein S) are the most commonly used after factor VIII. In addition, factor IX and factor XIII may be deficient in patients and are therefore sometimes required. Prothrombin complex concentrate contains factor II, factor V and factor X and is available from commercial sources for patients who are bleeding due to deficiency of these factors. The clinical requirements for their use are similar to those described earlier; for example, acquired coagulation factor deficiency or liver disease will result in multiple clotting deficiencies which may be treated by factor concentrates. Haemophilia B, or Christmas disease, is a congenital deficiency of factor IX and requires regular infusion of factor IX concentrate to prevent haemorrhage and bruising.

Fresh frozen plasma and cryoprecipitate

These components differ in that they are usually produced from single donations from which the plasma has been removed and frozen quickly. **Fresh frozen plasma** (FFP) is rich in coagulation factors. Coagulation factors undergo various degrees of deterioration, especially when not kept frozen. Plasma (platelet-poor) is removed from the red cells within 6 hours of the blood being donated, frozen rapidly at $-70°C$, and stored at $-30°C$ to maintain the coagulation factors at optimum levels.

Coagulation deficiencies or haemorrhage can occur in many clinical situations. Some examples are massive blood loss, infection or surgery to the liver (which is usually the site of synthesis for clotting factors), and acquired multiple coagulation factor deficiencies. It is usual for a patient to be infused with 1 litre of FFP at a time and for the clinical benefit to be checked by coagulation tests in the laboratory. Recipients of fresh frozen plasma should be issued ABO group specific donated plasma to prevent a transfusion reaction due to anti-A or anti-B (see Chapter 5 for antibodies present in plasma). Fresh frozen plasma may be virally inactivated using chemical treatment with methylene blue in order to ensure the safety of the product regarding disease transmission.

Cryoprecipitate is a source of factor VIII extracted from the plasma of single donors. It has been extensively used for the treatment of haemophiliacs for many years but is now less often used, as viral-inactivated factor VIII concentrate is widely available. Cryoprecipitate was discovered by Pool and Shannon in 1965 and is formed, as the name suggests, by the precipitation of a fraction of the plasma which is enriched with factor VIII when frozen and then slowly thawed. This process must take place within a few hours of blood collection as factor VIII has a half-life of just a few hours at room temperature. Cryoprecipitate is also a source of fibrinogen and is sometimes used for patients with low plasma levels of this protein.

Platelet concentrates

Platelets are normally formed in the bone marrow and released into the circulation where they have a role in haemostasis. Platelets clump together, or aggregate, in response to substances produced when damage to the blood vessel lining has occurred. This forms a platelet plug, which has the effect of preventing blood loss from the damaged vessel wall. The coagulation system is also activated to form fibrin and a platelet–fibrin thrombus results. Patients who are lacking in platelets are therefore prone to bruising due to small haemorrhages into the tissues, and bleeding, for example nose bleeds (epistaxis). This condition is known as **thrombocytopenia**. Low numbers of circulating platelets may be due to disease, particularly leukaemia and aplastic anaemia. Drug treatment, such as the use of cytotoxic drugs which affect the haemopoietic (blood-producing) cells in the bone marrow, can give rise to the condition, and bone marrow transplant patients are also thrombocytopenic. Patients requiring massive transfusion or heart–lung bypass surgery are likely to have a low circulating platelet count due to dilution. Inherited disorders of platelet function are sometimes detected and these patients require platelet transfusions to prevent haemorrhage.

The transfusion of platelet concentrates is an effective way of raising the circulating platelet numbers. The normal platelet count is $150–400 \times 10^9 \, l^{-1}$; levels may fall to as low as less than $5 \times 10^9 \, l^{-1}$ and a number of units of platelet concentrate may be required to raise the levels to at least $20 \times 10^9 \, l^{-1}$. The effectiveness is established in the laboratory by checking the platelet count pre- and post-transfusion. As the survival of platelets is approximately 10 days, and in transfused platelets this is reduced to 4 days, regular transfusions are needed.

Platelet concentrates are prepared by two methods. Firstly, donated blood is subjected to a slow centrifugation in which the platelets, having a relatively low density, settle in the upper plasma layer. The platelet-rich plasma is then aspirated into a 'satellite' plastic pack and further centrifuged to sediment the platelets into a concentrate in a small volume of plasma. The upper layer of platelet-poor plasma is aspirated and used for further fractionation. The second method is by **plasmapheresis** using a cell separator. This technique involves the removal of donor blood by insertion of a catheter into a vein; as the blood enters the cell separator selective centrifugation takes place at a speed which removes the platelets. The remaining platelet-depleted blood is returned to the donor via a catheter inserted into a vein in the other arm. This method results in a higher yield of platelets (at least $3.0 \times 10^{11} \, l^{-1}$ compared to $5.5 \times 10^{10} \, l^{-1}$ from the whole blood donor method), though there is more contamination with leukocytes than with the whole blood donor technique (see the problems associated with leukocytes discussed earlier). Whichever technique is used, the subsequent conditions in which the platelets are kept prior to transfusion are important. The physiological role of platelets is to become activated in response to trauma and this must be avoided so that the platelets can still be effective in platelet plug formation once they are transfused. It has been found that platelets are best stored at 22°C with continuous gentle movement, as provided by placing on an 'agitator'. The shelf-life of platelets is 5 days. Platelets for newborn infants may be prepared using the technique of apheresis as well as single donor sources. The donated platelets can then be split into four smaller units for transfusion to the infant. Further procedures are also required for neonates, such as removal of the white cells, selecting a CMV negative donor and screening extensively to exclude the presence of antibodies.

Quality assurance

All products derived from blood are subjected to rigorous quality control procedures by blood centres and the Bio-Products Laboratory in the UK. Component processing must comply with the regulations and standards of Good Manufacturing Practice and Good Pharmaceutical Practice as appropriate. It is necessary to ensure that the product contains adequate levels of the component stated on its label, and also that it is processed and stored correctly from manufacture to the issuing of the product to the hospital and finally to the patient at the bedside. The prevention of disease transmission by blood components is highly significant since the advent of the human immunodeficiency virus (HIV) and more recently the uncertainties surrounding the transmission of the bovine spongiform encephalitis related scrapie virus which in humans causes new variant Creutzfeldt-Jakob disease. Further discussion of disease transmission by blood products and components can be found in Chapter 10.

Suggested further reading

Contreras, M., ed. (1996). *ABC of Transfusion*. London: BMJ
   Publishing Group.
Barbara, J. and Flanagan, P. (1998). Blood transfusion risk:
   protecting against the unknown. *British Medical Journal*, **316**,
   part 7133, 717–718.

Self-assessment questions

1. List the components of whole blood for transfusion.
2. Give examples of clinical cases where red cell transfusion may
   be needed.
3. Describe the optimal conditions for the storage of platelets.
4. What is the role of 2,3-diphosphoglycerate (2,3-DPG) in red
   cells?
5. Give reasons why the presence of leukocytes in a transfusion
   may be of risk to the patient.
6. List the methods that are currently available to inactivate or
   remove viruses in blood products and components.

Key Concepts and Facts

- Blood for transfusion is separated into red cells and plasma/
  plasma-derived components.

- Blood and blood components are valuable in treating a variety
  of diseases and disorders.

- Blood and blood components must be anticoagulated and
  stored in an appropriate manner to be effective when transfused to a patient.

- Blood is a source of infection and a number of procedures are
  required to minimize the risk of disease transmission.

- Quality assurance procedures are an essential part of blood
  product and component therapy.

Chapter 9
Haemagglutination and blood grouping methods

Learning objectives

After studying this chapter you should confidently be able to:

Describe the two stages of haemagglutination.

Describe the forces involved in antibody binding.

Discuss the forces involved in the formation of agglutinates.

List the methods available for overcoming zeta potential.

List the various ways of visualizing haemagglutination reactions.

Describe the nature and control of the antiglobulin test.

List the causes of false agglutination test results.

Traditionally the visualization of red cell antigen/antibody reactions in the laboratory is achieved by either haemagglutination (or its inhibition) or haemolysis of red cells. Complement-mediated haemolysis is not particularly common with red cell antibodies; most do not fix sufficient complement to progress to lysis (see Chapter 3 for more details). More usually complement is activated to the C3b stage, at which point natural inhibitors and inactivators stop the reaction resulting in degradation of the C3 molecule to leave cell-bound C3dg. This degradation product is then detected by agglutination brought about by anti-C3d reagents.

Agglutination techniques developed over many years have proved to be robust and (deceptively) simple to perform. The physicochemical factors involved in agglutination, however, are much more complex. Transfusion scientists need to have a thorough understanding of the factors involved in haemagglutination to be able to appreciate fully how variations in reaction conditions can affect test results. It is also important in order to be able to make informed judgements on new or variant methodologies. Experience is also required to differentiate true agglutination from other phenomena which may cause 'clumping' of red cells, e.g. fibrin clots, rouleaux, comets, and red cell adherence to dust and dirt.

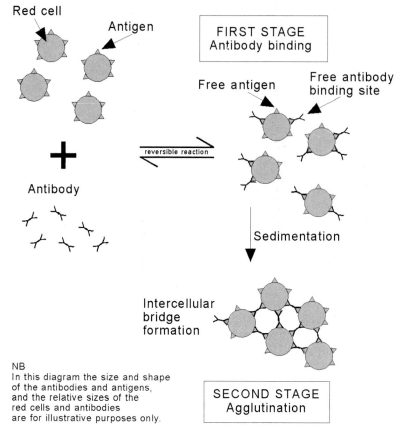

Figure 9.1   *Diagrammatic representation of the first and second stages of haemagglutination*

Haemagglutination

Haemagglutination occurs in two stages. In the first stage red cell antibodies attach to their corresponding antigen. Various terms have been used to describe this stage, such as binding, sensitization, association or coating. In the second stage intercellular bridges are formed as the free combining sites on the attached red cell antibodies bind to free antigen sites on adjacent red cells. The lattice thus formed is termed an agglutinate (see Figure 9.1).

First stage of agglutination (binding of antibody)

The antibody combining sites of immunoglobulins (Fab) are complementary in shape and charge to the antigens with which they react, enabling them to come into close contact and allowing the formation of reversible bonds (see Chapter 2). Several forces and types of bond are involved in this process of antibody binding.

- **Ionic bonds** are formed by the transfer of electrons from donor to acceptor ionic and non-ionic groups between the antibody and its antigen. This electrostatic force of attraction is inversely proportional to the square of the distance separating the charged surfaces of the red cells and antibodies. This results in a rapid increase in the magnitude of the force as the antigen and antibody surfaces approach one another. The levels of ionization and charge on the antigen and antibody depend significantly on the pH of the immediate environment.

- **Hydrophobic bonds** arise from the tendency of non-polar groups to avoid water and adhere to one another. The amino acids alanine, leucine, isoleucine, phenylalanine and tryptophan all provide free non-polar groups for hydrophobic bonding in most protein molecules.

- **Hydrogen bonds** arise from the reaction between hydrogen atoms that are covalently bound to strongly electronegative atoms (such as oxygen and nitrogen) and unshared electron pairs of other electronegative atoms. This is due to the relative electropositivity of the hydrogen nucleus. Hydrogen bonding is primarily exothermic in nature and so is further driven by reduced temperatures. This is known as Le Chatelier's principle.

- **van der Waal's forces** develop from the movement of electrons, which produces a general attraction of molecules over short distances. The force increases with increasing mass of the reactive sites and is inversely proportional to the seventh power of the distance separating the surfaces. This means that the antigen and antibody surfaces must come into close contact for these forces to be significant in antigen/antibody binding.

- **Randomization of water** occurs as water is squeezed out when antigen and antibody surfaces come together. This causes an increase in entropy, reduces competition with hydrogen bonds, lowers the dielectric constant around polar sites and increases the attractive free energy. These are all factors which favour the binding of antigen and antibody.

Antigen/antibody reactions are dependent on both thermal (enthalpy) and disorder (entropy) factors. As the antigen/antibody complexes approach equilibrium, entropy is maximized. In addition ionic bonds, hydrophobic bonds, hydrogen bonds and van der Waals forces affect all reactions to some extent. Thus the final antigen/antibody bond results from numerous types of physical forces as well as complementarity of shape and charge.

The bonds formed between antigen and antibody are reversible and may be expressed in terms of a mass action relationship. See Chapter 2 for a discussion of the binding affinity of antibodies.

Being a reversible thermodynamic reaction, this binding of antibody to antigen is affected by several factors:

- **Temperature.** Reduction in reaction temperature will reduce the rate of antibody association and disassociation but not necessarily the equilibrium affinity constant, K, which in some cases may be increased at lower temperatures. Increases in temperature will increase the rates of association and disassociation, but eventually a temperature will be reached where antibody is disassociating rather than associating (K reduced). Those antibodies which react best at lower temperatures (e.g. ABO, P_1) probably depend to a larger extent on exothermic hydrogen bonds for much of their strength of attachment.

- **pH**. The optimum range for antibody/antigen reactions is usually quoted as pH 6.5–6.8 with little effect in binding noted over the range pH 5.5–8.5. Some anti-D antibodies show reduced binding at higher pH and some anti-M antibodies show increased binding at lower pH. Generally, reduction in pH increases the complementarity of charges between antigen and antibody. This pH effect refers to the pH of the final reaction mixture, not the pH of individual reactants. The student's attention is drawn to the common practice of washing and suspending red cells in phosphate buffer solution with a pH of around 6.8–7.2. Apart from not being the optimum pH range for antibody/antigen reactions, it may be unnecessary due to the fact that both plasma and red cells act as very efficient buffers.

- **Ionic strength**. Physiological 'normal' saline used in blood group serology is a 0.85–0.9% solution of sodium chloride in water, with an ionic strength of $0.15\,mol\,l^{-1}$. Reduction in the ionic strength of the reaction medium (typically to $0.09\,mol\,l^{-1}$) increases the rate at which antibody binds to antigen (but not necessarily the amount bound at equilibrium). In normal saline the mobility of individual ions is restricted by the presence of so many other ions. In low ionic strength solutions (LISS) ions are generally able to be more mobile and this favours ionic bonding between antigen and antibody. In addition, the ionized groups on antigens and antibodies in saline will be partially neutralized by all the free ions in the solution, thus interfering with antigen/antibody binding. In LISS, this neutralization effect is much reduced. Reducing the ionic strength of the reaction medium by too great a factor facilitates the aggregation of normal serum globulins and their non-specific adhesion to red cells. This may lead to the activation and fixing of complement to the red cell. Subsequent washing of the red cells will remove the globulins but complement may stay attached to the cell and lead to a false positive reaction if the cells are tested with an anti-complement containing reagent such as polyspecific anti-human globulin reagent (see later).

- **Antigen and antibody concentration**. An increase in the concentration of reactants will favour the association reaction in the first stage of agglutination. However, this increase may reduce resultant agglutinate formation in the second stage and therefore its detection in the laboratory (see later in this section). There is a delicate balance in the relative concentrations of antigen and antibody, which needs to be achieved for optimal agglutination.

Second stage of agglutination (intercellular bridge formation)

This stage involves the formation of intercellular bridges between free binding sites on red cell bound antibodies and free antigen sites on adjacent red cells. There are three major factors affecting this stage: the forces of aggregation, the forces of repulsion and the relative concentrations of antigen and antibody.

Aggregating forces

Every surface has a certain amount of associated energy (for example X ergs cm^{-2}). When aggregation or agglutination of red cells takes place, two surfaces, each of a specific surface area, for example A cm^2, come into contact. The amount of energy held by these two surfaces, $2AX$ ergs, is also lost. The second law of thermodynamics states that a system is in equilibrium when its free energy is at a minimum. Thus the red cell surface tension acts in such a way as to produce aggregation in order to lose surface energy.

Repulsive forces

The most important force which opposes the aggregating effects of surface tension results from the electrical charge of the red cell membrane. The charge arises largely from the ionization of carboxyl groups of surface sialic acid residues carried on the glycophorins. This gives the membrane a net electronegative charge. The red cell surface potential charge is approximately -34 mV. As each red cell is equally charged, both in sign and magnitude, there exists between them a repulsive force which is inversely proportional to the square of the distance separating them (Coulomb's law). It is this repulsive force which prevents red cells adhering to vessel walls or to one another. The repulsive force exerted when the flatter surfaces of two red cells come together can be 10 times greater than when two curved surfaces come together. Thus highly curved surfaces can approach each other much more closely than flat surfaces (see Figure 9.2).

In the presence of electrolyte, such as sodium (or potassium) ions in plasma or saline, each red cell is surrounded by a cloud of oppositely charged ions (cations). The cloud decreases in density with increasing distance from the red cell surface. Part of this cloud of cations will move with the red cell and form part of its kinetic unit. The line of demarcation separating the cations which move with the red cell from the remaining cations in the medium is known as the **slipping plane** (see Figure 9.3).

> To help visualize the relative differences in size between antibody molecules and red cells, consider this comparison. If a red cell was 1 m in diameter then the maximum distance between binding sites for an IgM molecule would be approximately 4 mm and for an IgG molecule approximately 1.5 mm.

Figure 9.2   *Diagram showing the mutual repulsion between electronegative red cells*

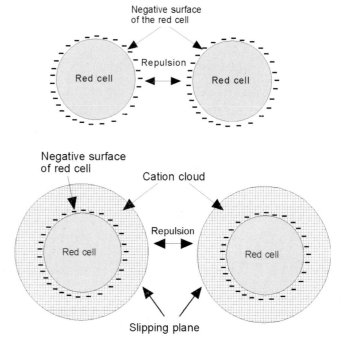

Figure 9.3   *Diagram showing red cells suspended in saline. Each red cell is surrounded by a cloud of cations (Na$^+$)*

It is convenient to consider this system as analogous to the charges on two concentric spheres (see Figure 9.4). The inner sphere corresponds to the red cell surface and the outer represents the slipping plane of the cation cloud. The net charge density of the cation cloud is greater than that at the red cell surface. The sum of the electrical potentials related to these two charged surfaces will determine the total voltage that acts through the space between the two spheres and appears as the potential at the surface of the outer sphere. It follows that the force of repulsion between two red cells is not dependent on the value of the charge or potential at the red cell surface, but rather on the potential that exists at the boundary which marks the slipping plane. This potential is known as the **zeta**

Figure 9.4   *Red cells surrounded by cations, represented as two concentric spheres. The inner sphere represents the electronegative surface of the red cell. The outer sphere represents the slipping plane of the electropositive cation cloud. The sum of the electrical potentials related to these two surfaces determines the total voltage that acts through the space between the two spheres and appears as the potential at the surface of the outer sphere. This is the zeta potential*

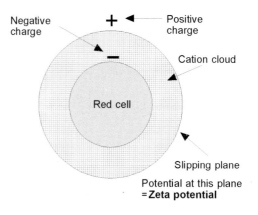

potential (Figure 9.4). Its magnitude will depend on the volume net charge density of the surrounding cations, i.e. the ionic strength of the medium.

The zeta potential for red cells suspended in normal saline is approximately −18 mV. At this value the repulsive forces keep the red cells apart by around 18–20 nm. In order for an antibody to bring about direct agglutination of saline-suspended cells (sometimes called a complete antibody) it would have to span the 20 nm gap between adjacent cells. IgM antibodies have a maximum distance between binding sites of around 30 nm and so can readily span the gap between red cells. IgG antibodies have a maximum distance between binding sites of around 12 nm and so cannot usually bring about the direct agglutination of saline-suspended red cells (sometimes known as incomplete antibodies; see Figure 9.5). However, if the antigen protrudes some distance from the cell surface, even IgG antibodies may be able to effect direct agglutination, as the distance between their target antigens would be less than the distance between the red cell surfaces. For example, ABO antigens may protrude from the cell surface by as much as 5 nm. Although the distance between adjacent cell surfaces is 20 nm, the distance between ABO antigens may therefore be as little as 10 nm. At this distance IgG anti-A or anti-B would be able to attach to antigens on adjacent cells and so bring about direct agglutination.

The value of the zeta potential may be reduced in order to allow the closer approach of red cells by either increasing the ionic strength or the dielectric constant of the suspending medium, or by decreasing the charge at the red cell surface.

- **Ionic strength.** As can be seen from the formula shown (see sidebox), an increase in ionic strength will reduce the zeta potential as more cations are packed around the red cell, increasing the density of the cation cloud and neutralizing more of the red cell surface charge. As described in the earlier section on factors affecting the first stage of agglutination, increasing the

---

For human red cells at 25°C the zeta potential may be represented by the following formula:

$$\text{Zeta potential} = \frac{4.27}{D\mu}$$
$$+ \frac{309}{D} \text{ mV}$$

where D = the dielectric constant of the medium and μ = the ionic strength of the medium. Red cells have a zeta potential of approximately −34 mV which is reduced to −18 mV when the red cells are suspended in normal saline. The **critical zeta** for an antibody is the value above which the antibody cannot bring about direct agglutination (because the red cells are held too far apart). For IgM (complete) antibodies this value is around −23 mV and for IgG (incomplete) antibodies it is around −13 mV.

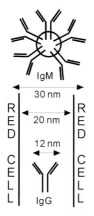

Figure 9.5 *Diagram illustrating the distance between red cells suspended in normal saline. The IgG antibody molecules are too small to span the gap between adjacent red cells (incomplete antibody), whereas the IgM antibody molecules are large enough to span the gap and bring about direct agglutination (complete antibody)*

ionic strength will decrease the amount of antibody able to bind to antigen. This inhibition of antibody binding limits the usefulness of this method for reducing zeta potential. Students often fail to understand that **decreasing the ionic strength will cause an increase in zeta potential and thus force red cells even further apart** than in normal saline. Another way to visualize this is that, as there are less ions available to neutralize red cell surface charge, there will be greater repulsion between cells. The use of a low ionic strength solution (LISS) technique, then, is inappropriate for the detection of antibodies by direct agglutination. This should be noted and considered in laboratory tests.

- **Dielectric constant.** This is a measure of the charge dissipating properties of a substance. As can be seen from the formula shown, an increase in dielectric constant will reduce the zeta potential. Certain water-soluble polymers, such as albumin, polyvinyl pyrrolidine and dextran, will raise the dielectric constant of water by an amount that is dependent upon the degree to which they become polarized and oriented in an electric field. In effect they have areas of their molecule which can be either positively or negatively charged. Thus, unlike simple ions, they are both attracted and repelled by the red cell surface charge. They are therefore forced to orientate themselves or rotate in such a way that they are less randomly distributed in the medium. The energy required for this polarization is obtained from the electric field surrounding the red cell and so the zeta potential is reduced.

- **Red cell surface charge.** Reducing the electrical charge at the red cell surface will obviously reduce the repulsive forces and so allow the closer approach of cells. This reduction in charge is usually brought about with the use of proteolytic enzymes such as papain, bromelin and ficin. The enzymes are used to remove red cell surface proteins expressing sialic acid residues which contribute the majority of the cell's negative charge.

The **use of enzymes** can also enhance antigen/antibody reactions in a number of other ways:

- The enzymes may reveal new antigens or make hidden antigen sites more accessible as surface proteins are removed from the cell.

- They may increase the mobility of protein within the red cell membrane. This allows the clustering of antigen which in turn allows the formation of multiple, adjacent intercellular bridges, thus enhancing agglutination.

- They reduce hydration at the red cell surface, which favours antigen/antibody binding.

- They promote the production of irregular protrusions from the red cells. These protrusions have highly curved surfaces and therefore exhibit less repulsive force, allowing red cells to approach more closely.

The surface charge may also be reduced by the binding of antibodies on to the red cell. The degree of reduction is dependent on the amount of antibody bound and the charges covered. Usually the reduction in charge and resultant reduction in zeta potential is less than 25% of the initial value. However, if sufficient IgG antibody is bound then a (usually) incomplete IgG antibody may cause direct agglutination of saline-suspended cells. For example, cells of the rare Rh phenotype D−− (see Chapter 5) express very large amounts of Rh D antigen and therefore bind large amounts of anti-D antibody. The red cell surface charge may be reduced to such an extent that the cells are agglutinated in saline suspension with an otherwise incomplete antibody.

As mentioned earlier, reducing the ionic strength of the reaction medium too much facilitates the aggregation of normal serum globulins and their non-specific adhesion to red cells. This can cause a considerable reduction in surface charge and lead to non-antibody mediated red cell aggregation, which cannot be distinguished from true agglutination.

The effect of the zeta potential may be overcome in several other ways, as outlined below.

- **Action of macromolecules**. In addition to increasing the dielectric constant of the reaction medium, macromolecules may facilitate agglutination by: (i) bringing about large areas of cell to cell contact by physical adhesion (polymer bridging) of the red cells – this allows for the formation of multiple, adjacent intercellular antigen/antibody bridges; (ii) reducing hydration and thus increasing attractive free energy around antigen/antibody binding sites; (iii) increasing extracellular colloid osmotic pressure which may induce red cell shape changes – these shape changes may allow for larger areas of cell to cell contact brought about by polymer bridging.

- **Action of polycationic polymers**. Polycationic polymers are substances, such as polybrene, which express multiple electro-positive regions. They can readily bring about the aggregation of electronegative particles, including red cells. They facilitate agglutination by: (i) aggregating red cells and thus bringing them closer together to allow the formation of intercellular antigen/antibody bridges; (ii) facilitating large areas of cell to cell contact via polymer bridging (see above); (iii) reducing hydration and thus increasing attractive free energy around antigen/antibody binding sites; (iv) inducing red cell shape changes – these shape changes may allow for larger areas of cell to cell contact brought about by polymer bridging.

- **Spiculation**. This is the formation of long protrusions from the red cell membrane. Such protrusions will have highly curved points and so exhibit less repulsion than flat surfaces. This allows for closer cell to cell contact. ABO antibodies in particular have been demonstrated to induce spiculation when binding to red cells.

Concentration of antigen and antibody

Increases in the concentration of antigen or antibody will favour binding in stage one of agglutination. However, the formation of agglutinates will be inhibited if the relative concentrations of antigen to antibody are not optimized.

- **Excess antigen**. Conditions of relative excess of antigen in a reaction mixture include the use of too strong a red cell suspension, the addition of too small a volume of serum, the addition of too large a volume of cell suspension and low levels of antibody in the serum. Under these conditions antibodies will be so thinly distributed amongst the red cells that the formation of intercellular bridges will be sparse and only involve small numbers of cells (see Figure 9.6).

- **Excess antibody**. Conditions of relative excess of antibody in a reaction mixture include the use of too weak a cell suspension, cells expressing small numbers of antigen sites, the addition of too large a volume of serum, the addition of too small a volume of cell suspension and high levels of antibody in the serum. Under these conditions the majority of antigen sites will be coated with antibody, leaving few free antigen sites available for attachment to the free binding sites on antibodies attached to adjacent red cells. Thus there is a reduction in intercellular bridge formation and corresponding agglutination (see Figure 9.7).

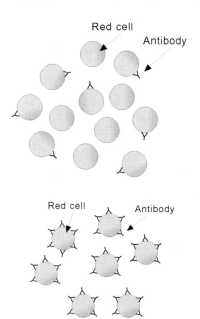

Figure 9.6 *Diagrammatic representation of conditions of relative excess of antigen. The antibody is so sparsely distributed that few opportunities for intercellular bridge formation exist*

Figure 9.7 *Diagrammatic representation of conditions of relative excess of antibody. Most antigen sites are coated with antibody so that there are too few free antigen sites available on adjacent cells for the formation of intercellular bridges*

Methods

It is beyond the scope of this text to give detailed procedures for carrying out the large number of haemagglutination techniques currently available. Instead this section gives an overview of techniques and practical considerations and relates them to the various factors involved in haemagglutination.

Direct agglutination

Red cells suspended in saline are kept apart, due to mutual repulsion, by a distance of approximately 20 nm. Direct agglutination of red cells suspended in saline is usually only observed with IgM antibodies, which are large enough to span the gap between adjacent cells. For this agglutination to occur, however, the correct balance of antigen and antibody concentration must be achieved. Many years of practical experience have demonstrated that most direct agglutination reactions are optimized by mixing equal volumes of serum and a 3% suspension of red cells in saline.

Direct agglutination of red cells by IgG antibodies may be brought about by using techniques that reduce the electrical repulsion between red cells (zeta potential), allowing them to come into closer contact. Such techniques usually have other advantages such as encouraging multiple intercellular antibody bridge formation (polymer bridging, antigen clustering, red cell shape changes), reducing the degree of hydration at the red cell surface which favours antigen/antibody binding and, in the case of enzymes, making antigen sites more accessible to their corresponding antibodies. It should be remembered that techniques which allow direct agglutination by IgG antibodies may also enhance the action of IgM antibodies.

Techniques that have been commonly used to bring about direct agglutination by IgG antibodies are outlined below.

Use of albumin

Usually 20–30% bovine serum albumin is used or high molecular weight polymers which reduce zeta potential by raising the dielectric constant of the reaction medium. This dissipates the charge surrounding the red cells and allows closer contact of the cells. Several variations of albumin techniques exist:

- **Displacement or replacement** methods, in which albumin is added towards the end of the reaction incubation period after the red cells have settled into a button in the tube. The high density albumin either displaces or replaces the supernatant serum and saline to leave the cells in an albumin-rich (high dielectric constant) environment for the remainder of the incubation period.

Some technical factors affecting haemagglutination reactions are listed below.

- **Reagent volumes**. The volumes dispensed must be accurate and reproducible to avoid excesses of antigen or antibody. If a Pasteur or dropper pipette is being used it must be held at the same angle for the dispensing of all reagents. A pipette held towards the horizontal relative to the test tube will dispense significantly larger volumes than a pipette held towards the vertical. Static electrical charge on the test tubes (a particular problem with plastic tubes) may affect the volume of the drop dispensed from a pipette by 'dragging' extra reagent from the tip of the pipette or by deflecting the drops as they approach the mouth of the test tube. Static may be dispersed by standing racks of tubes in a water-bath for a few seconds prior to use.

- **Cell concentrations**. Accurate concentrations of red cell suspensions are important to avoid relative excesses of antigen (cell suspension too strong) or antibody (cell suspension too weak). Most transfusion scientists learn by experience to judge commonly used cell concentrations 'by eye'.

- **Mixing reactants**. Thorough mixing of red cells and serum in the test tube is important (except in layering techniques) to allow maximum contact between antibodies and red cells.

- **Zoning**. A serum containing a relative excess of antibody may not bring about direct agglutination until it has been diluted to the point where the optimum concentration of antigen and antibody is achieved. Further dilution of the serum leads to reducing degrees of agglutination as would normally be expected. This

- **Albumin suspension** methods, in which the red cells are suspended in an albumin solution instead of saline from the beginning of the test.
- **Layering** methods, in which typing or test serum is layered on to a cell button at the beginning of the test. The serum itself then provides the high protein environment for the test.

Albumin techniques are generally not as sensitive as some of the other techniques available for detecting IgG antibodies. In addition there can be great variation between batches of albumin and the tests may be difficult to read due to stickiness and comet formation (see later). For these reasons albumin techniques are no longer commonly used for antibody screening, although they may be useful in characterizing some antibodies.

Use of proteolytic enzymes

Proteolytic enzymes such as papain, bromelin and ficin can be used to reduce red cell surface charge by removing proteins (particularly glycophorins) carrying electronegative sialic acid residues. Several variations are in common use, using either a one- or two-stage procedure.

In **one-stage methods** red cells, enzyme and serum are mixed together in the same tube. There are three basic variations within this methodology:

- The **one-stage mix** method, which involves the simultaneous addition of cells, enzyme and antibody. This method has the disadvantages that the enzyme will also degrade the antibodies and some normal sera contain naturally occurring inhibitors of proteolytic enzymes.
- **Delay methods**, in which the red cells and enzyme are incubated together for a short time before the addition of the serum.
- **Inhibitor methods**, in which red cells and enzyme are incubated together for a short time and then an enzyme inhibitor is added before the addition of serum.

In **two-stage methods** the red cells are pre-treated with enzyme, washed and then reacted with serum.

Enzyme techniques are generally very good for the detection of Rh antibodies but, as the enzymes destroy MN and Duffy antigens, cannot be used to detect antibodies in these systems. Enzyme treatment of red cells is quite difficult to standardize and excessive treatment can lead to such a large reduction in surface charge that the cells spontaneously aggregate. It is also common to find clinically insignificant auto- and pan-antibodies (acting with all cells), reactive only with enzyme-treated cells. One-stage enzyme techniques have been shown to be much less reliable and less sensitive than two-stage techniques. The use of enzyme-treated cells can be a very useful tool in the characterization of a red cell antibody, but is generally no longer recommended for use as a screening technique.

Use of polycationic polymers

Polycationic polymers such as polybrene cause aggregation of electronegative red cells and so bring them into close contact. Typically, red cells and serum are incubated in a low ionic strength environment (to accelerate antibody binding), then polybrene is added to aggregate the cells and bring them into close contact. The non-specific aggregation is then dispersed by the addition of sodium citrate, but any antibody-mediated agglutination will remain. Polybrene techniques are rapid, good for the detection of Rh antibodies and do not suffer from the large number of unwanted positive results found with enzyme techniques. However, the detection rate for Kell, Duffy and Lewis antibodies can be particularly poor. For this reason, such techniques cannot be recommended for use as a stand-alone antibody screening method.

Chemical modification

The chemical modification of IgG molecules constitutes a some-what different approach to the problem of IgG molecules being too small to bridge the gap between red cells suspended in saline. The distance between the antigen binding sites (Fab) on an IgG antibody can be increased by chemical reduction of the disulphide bonds in the hinge region. Using this technique it has proved to be possible to produce stable IgG antibodies capable of spanning the distance between adjacent red cells suspended in saline. This approach lends itself to the production of typing sera but has no practical application in the detection of antibodies in the sera of patients.

Indirect agglutination

The antiglobulin test (AGT) was described in 1945 by Coombs *et al.* and was originally called the Coombs test. It remains the single most important test for IgG antibody detection and identification. In the AGT the binding of IgG antibody to red cells is visualized indirectly by the addition of **anti-human globulin (AHG)** reagent, containing antibodies to human IgG, to complete the intercellular bridging required for visible haemagglutination. The AGT may be performed directly on patients' red cells to detect *in vivo* binding of antibody (the direct antiglobulin test or **DAT**) or may be performed on cells that have been incubated with antibody *in vitro* (the indirect antiglobulin test or **IAT**). In both cases the AHG will bind to red cell bound IgG antibodies on adjacent red cells and bring about agglutination by a red cell–antibody–AHG–antibody–

Figure 9.8 *Diagrammatic representation of agglutination in the antiglobulin test. The red cells are too far apart for the IgG antibodies to cause direct agglutination. The addition of the anti-human globulin (AHG) reagent containing anti-IgG antibodies brings about agglutination by attaching to the red cell bound IgG molecules and forming cell–IgG–anti-IgG–IgG–cell intercellular bridges. All free IgG must be washed away before the addition of the AHG reagent to prevent binding of the anti-IgG to free IgG rather than cell-bound IgG*

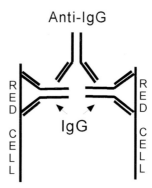

In the early 1940s R.R.A. Coombs was a research worker in the Department of Pathology at Cambridge University. He became interested in the nature of incomplete Rh antibodies after a discussion over coffee one day with R.R. Race. At that time it was not known whether these incomplete antibodies were true globulin antibodies. Together they demonstrated that incomplete Rh antibody was indeed a globulin antibody. They then went on to consider a test to demonstrate more easily these incomplete antibodies. It was in 1945, whilst travelling from London to Cambridge on a late night, badly lit train, that Coombs, deep in thought, visualized the antibody on the red cell and how it might be detected using antibody to serum globulin. The basic idea for this most important of all red cell serology tests, the **Coombs (antiglobulin) test**, had been born.

red cell bridge. This intercellular bridge is much greater in size than the distance between adjacent red cells (see Figure 9.8).

In direct agglutination techniques, relative excesses of antigen or antibody must be avoided in order to maximize the agglutination. This is not the case with the AGT and the ratio of antibody to antigen (serum to cells) may be increased to allow more antibody to bind and thus increase the sensitivity of the test. Typically serum to cell ratios of 70 : 1 or more are used. This is double the ratio found in standard direct agglutination tests. It is the AHG reagent which brings about the eventual agglutination and this reagent must therefore be standardized to give optimal agglutination at the desired serum to cell ratio.

Most modern AHG reagents are polyspecific. That is, they contain a blend of polyclonal anti-IgG (anti-human IgG produced in animals) and a monoclonal anti-C3d. The anti-IgG component brings about the agglutination of IgG coated cells as described above. The anti-C3d component is itself an IgM antibody and so brings about the direct agglutination of red cells coated with the stable complement fraction, C3dg (see Chapter 3), which may be attached to red cells by the action of some clinically significant IgG or IgM antibodies. The classic AGT requires a wash phase to remove any free globulin which would otherwise neutralize the AHG reagent. IgM antibodies are particularly prone to being washed from red cells during this phase of the test and so it is more reliable to detect the complement fixed to the cell by the IgM than to try to detect the IgM antibody itself. In addition, many hundreds of molecules of complement may be fixed to the red cell by each IgM molecule, and so detecting complement is a simpler and more sensitive test.

In attempts to increase the sensitivity of antibody detection, many workers have devised variations of the AGT. The main variations are described briefly below.

Normal ionic strength antiglobulin test (NIS-AGT)

This test is closest to the original techniques in which, typically, four volumes of serum are mixed with one or two volumes of 3% red cells suspended in normal saline. The test is incubated at 37°C for 45–60 minutes prior to washing and addition of AHG regent.

Low ionic strength antiglobulin test (LIS-AGT)

The use of a low ionic strength medium increases the rate of antibody uptake on to the red cells and so incubation times are reduced to between 15 and 20 minutes. Low ionic strength solutions are solutions of low salt concentration with the addition of substances to maintain isotonic conditions, e.g. glycine. To preserve the low ionic strength conditions in the test, equal volumes of serum and cells suspended in low ionic strength medium must be used. This means that, in order to achieve a more sensitive serum to cell ratio, as in the NIS-AGT, the cell concentration has to be reduced to between 1.5 and 2%. Several variations of the LIS-AGT exist:

- **LIS suspension** methods, which utilize red cells suspended in a low ionic strength medium.
- **LIS additive** methods, which utilize the addition of a reagent to create the low ionic strength conditions.
- Use of **polyethylene glycol (PEG)** combined with a low ionic strength additive. PEG is a water-soluble polymer which has been shown to act as a potentiator of antigen/antibody reactions.
- The **low ionic strength polybrene** method (described in the section on direct agglutination), followed by washing of the red cells and addition of AHG.

The LIS-suspension method is the most common variation of the AGT in general use in the UK. As previously discussed, reducing the ionic strength can lead to the non-specific uptake of globulin and fixation of complement on to red cells, leading to false positive reactions. It is therefore usually recommended that LIS-AGTs are used with AHG reagents containing only anti-IgG. Many clinically insignificant antibodies which only react in the LIS-AGT (and not in the NIS-AGT) have been described. The detection of these antibodies can lead to delays in the provision of blood for transfusion whilst attempts are being made to identify the antibodies.

Absorption and elution

The **absorption of antibodies** from serum onto red cells is a procedure that may be used in a variety of situations:

- To remove unwanted antibody from a typing serum.
- To remove antibody from a serum containing a mixture of antibodies, to aid identification.

Since its original use, changes have been made to the anti-human globulin reagent. The original Coombs reagent typically contained:

- Anti-IgA
- Anti-IgG
- Anti-IgM
- Antibodies to several C3 and C4 complement fragments

Modern polyspecific AHG reagents contain:

- Anti-IgG
- Anti-C3d

- To detect the presence of weakly expressed antigens by their ability to absorb the corresponding antibody.

The section on the factors affecting antibody binding described how increasing the concentration of antigen increased the amount of antibody bound to the red cell. In practice this means adding a slight excess volume of concentrated red cells to a volume of serum from which the antibody is to be absorbed.

Antibody elution is a procedure for the removal and recovery of red cell bound antibody, into an inert medium, for subsequent identification. The inert medium containing the eluted antibody is known as the **eluate**.

Examples where the preparation of an eluate is required include:

- The identification of antibodies bound to patients' red cells *in vivo*, as in cases of autoimmune haemolytic anaemia or haemolytic disease of the newborn.
- The identification of antibodies bound to transfused red cells, particularly in cases of delayed transfusion reaction.
- The identification of antibodies absorbed on to red cells from a serum containing a mixture of antibodies.
- Demonstration of the presence of weak antigens on red cells by the elution of the corresponding antibody from those cells after performing antibody absorption as described above, e.g. the demonstration of weak subgroups of the A antigen.

There are several elution procedures in common use. Some utilize a modification of the factors affecting the binding of antibody to antigen, such as changes in pH, temperature or ionic strength, to remove the antibody. Others rely on physical disruption of the red cell membrane by solvents or freezing and thawing to release the bound antibody.

Technical considerations

Antiglobulin tests

As already explained, the AGT is the most important of all the methods available for the detection of clinically significant antibodies. Therefore the risk of false negative results in particular must be minimized. The two most common causes of a false negative AGT are inadequate washing of red cells prior to the addition of AHG and disruption of agglutinates by a poor technique for reading results.

Inadequate washing of red cells prior to the addition of AHG may leave sufficient residual serum globulin to neutralize the AHG reagent. Centrifuges used to wash cells need to be quality assured regularly to ensure thorough washing is occurring. All negative tests should be controlled by the addition of red cells pre-sensitized with

IgG antibody. If the control cells agglutinate then sufficient free AHG is available and the negative test results are valid. If the control cells do not agglutinate then it can be assumed that the AHG reagent has been neutralized by free serum globulin, due to inadequate washing. The negative test result in this case would be invalid and would require repeating. The pre-sensitized cells are coated in sufficient antibody to give a weak reaction with AHG. This makes them more sensitive for detecting partial neutralization of the AHG regent. Typically the sensitized control cells should detect the presence of serum globulin at a dilution of one part in 1000.

To avoid false negative results due to **poor reading technique**, laboratories should operate an internal quality assurance programme to regularly assess an individual worker's ability to read weakly positive AGTs.

Typing red cells with a positive DAT

The red cell phenotyping of patients who have a positive direct antiglobulin test (e.g. in autoimmune haemolytic anaemia or haemolytic disease of the newborn) can pose particular problems. As the red cells from these patients are already coated in antibody, any phenotyping test which involves the use of a high protein medium (e.g. albumin tests) or AHG may lead to a positive reaction irrespective of whether the cell is positive or not with respect to the typing serum. To accurately type such patients it is necessary to use a direct agglutinating, low protein reagent such as an IgM monoclonal typing serum.

A related problem may occur when typing the red cells of a baby suffering from HDNB. A false negative result may occur with a direct agglutinating typing serum if the antigen being tested for is completely masked (or blocked) by maternal antibody. For example, when attempting to Rh D type the cells from a baby with a positive DAT due to maternal anti-D, all the Rh D antigen sites on the baby's cells may already be coated with maternal antibody. They are not, therefore, available for reaction with the typing serum and the baby would type as Rh D negative. To confirm that the baby is Rh D positive, it is necessary to elute the antibody from the baby's red cells and identify it as anti-D.

Visualization of agglutination

Scoring of the strength of agglutination reactions can give valuable information about the antibody/antigen reaction. For instance, it will give clues concerning antibodies which show dosage reactions, or cells which express weaker or stronger forms of an antigen (see Table 9.1).

Phenomena that may be falsely interpreted as agglutination are listed below.

- **Clots**. Small blood clots involving red cells may be misread as agglutination. They usually have smooth edges, whereas agglutinates are ragged and irregular.

- **Rouleaux**. This is the aggregation of red cells on their flat surfaces such that they resemble piles of coins. They tend to be more regular in appearance than agglutinates and under the microscope usually refract light differently such that they appear more orange in colour, whereas agglutinates are dark. Rouleaux can often be dispersed by the addition of a drop of clean saline to the slide.

- **Comets**. Certain high protein techniques, such as those using albumin, cause red cells to stick together loosely. This can be differentiated from agglutination by the smooth edges and the observation that, when looking at a moving field, the sticky mass of red cells rolls along leaving a trail of free cells. In this way it resembles a comet with a tail.

- **Debris**. The irregular appearance of red cells adhering to debris on a slide may resemble true agglutination. By observing a moving field, the debris can usually be seen to be floating on the surface of the sample rather than within the sample, as is the case with agglutination.

Table 9.1 *Example of an agglutination scoring system*

Score	Agglutinates	Free cells
5+	Massive clumps	Very few
4+	Several large clumps	Some
3+	Many macroscopic clumps	More
2+	Clump of 10–20 cells	Many
1+	Small microscopic clumps	Background of free cells
0	None	All

Agglutination reactions can be performed in a variety of reaction vessels, such as test tubes, slides, microplates or microtubes. They may be read macroscopically, microscopically or with the aid of a photometer or image analysis system.

Reactions in test tubes require the red cells to be sedimented to form a button at the bottom of the tube. This is achieved either by gravity or gentle centrifugation. The cell button can then be examined for agglutination either macroscopically or microscopically. Agglutinates of red cells can be very fragile and must be handled gently. **Macroscopic examination**, which may involve the use of an optical aid such as a magnifying lens or mirror, may be achieved by:

- Resuspension of the cells using a gentle **tapping** action. This method is only advisable with the most avid antibodies such as monoclonal ABO and Rh typing sera.

- Observation of the **settling pattern and streaming** of the red cells as the tube is gently tipped. Irregular settling patterns with no streaming indicate a positive reaction, while smooth settling patterns and streaming of cells on tipping indicate a negative reaction.

- Using a **tip and roll technique** in which the tube is gently tipped and simultaneously rolled between the thumb and first finger to resuspend the cells whilst observing for agglutination. This technique is particularly useful for reading AGTs.

Microscopic examination of cell buttons for agglutination is probably the most accurate way of reading agglutination tests when used by an experienced worker. The cell button is removed using a pipette and transferred to a microscope slide for examination. It is best to observe the cells using a relatively low power, such as a $\times 10$ eyepiece with a $\times 10$ objective, and observe moving fields. This may be achieved by gently tipping the slide or microscope so that the cells flow across the field of view. In inexperienced hands the fragile red cell agglutinates can be easily disrupted by poor pipetting technique. Alternatively, the red cells can be gently resuspended using the tip and roll technique described above and then the contents of the tube tipped directly on to a microscope slide.

Reactions on slides require the direct mixing of red cells and serum on the slide. The tests require constant, gentle mixing by rotation of the slide, to allow maximum cell to cell contact for intercellular bridge formation. Slide tests are usually read macroscopically and are best used only for avid antibodies.

The use of microplates enables the dispensing of reagents and samples and the reading of reactions to be quite easily automated. Microplate tests use either liquid phase or solid phase techniques. Liquid phase tests are similar to tube tests except they are performed in the wells of the microplate. Solid phase tests require either red cells or antibody to be physically bound to the wells. As with tube tests, cells must be sedimented in the wells either by gravity or gentle centrifugation before being read macroscopically, by photometer or by an image analysis system.

Macroscopic examination, which may involve the use of an optical aid such as a magnifying mirror, may be achieved by:

- Resuspension of the cells using gentle **agitation** of the microplate. This method is only advisable with the most avid antibodies such as monoclonal ABO and Rh typing sera.

- Observation of the **settling pattern and streaming** of the red cells as the microplate is gently tipped. Irregular settling patterns with no streaming indicate a positive reaction, while smooth settling patterns and streaming of cells on tipping indicate a negative reaction.

- The **use of a photometer** to read the settling patterns, using either single point, dual point or multipoint scanning of the microplate wells.

- The **use of image analysis** systems which take a 'picture' of each well and compare it to reference 'pictures' of positive and negative settling patterns.

Several **microtube systems** (sometimes called card, cassette, column agglutination or gel tests) are also now available. All the systems consist of six narrow tubes, each with a larger reaction chamber at the top, moulded into a plastic cassette or card. The tubes contain a density gradient material which allows red cells but not serum to pass through. In addition, the tubes contain either Sephadex gel or microbeads to trap agglutinated cells physically, or a substance such as protein G, which has a high affinity for IgG antibody, to trap IgG coated red cells.

Cells and serum are incubated in the upper reaction chamber of the microtubes. After appropriate incubation the cards are centrifuged and the red cells pass though the density gradient and into the trapping medium. Alternatively, typing sera may be incorporated into the microtubes so that red cells can be typed by immediate centrifugation into the matrix containing the antiserum, where they may be agglutinated and trapped. Also, AHG may be incorporated in the microtubes. As the density gradient only allows red cells to pass down the microtube, it is not necessary to wash the cells prior to contact with the AHG. Once again the agglutinates or antibody-coated cells will be trapped whilst free cells pass through to form a layer at the bottom of the microtube.

Microtube tests may be read **macroscopically**. Once the tubes have been centrifuged the reactions are stable for many hours or even days and so may be read when convenient. The centrifuged cards may be kept for later inspection by another worker or a supervisor if the results require a second opinion. Alternatively, the reactions may be read by **an image analysis system** which takes a 'picture' of each microtube and compares it to reference 'pictures' of positive and negative reaction patterns.

Associated considerations

Enhancement of reactions

Every enhancement method for detecting antigen/antibody reactions (e.g. LISS, polybrene, enzymes) and each preservative and additive has associated with it examples of false or unwanted positive reactions or false negative reactions. The unwanted positive reactions are usually due to clinically insignificant antibodies only detectable with a particular technique or in the presence of a particular preservative. Well reported examples include clinically insignificant antibodies reacting only in LIS-AGTs, antibodies which react only in the presence of EDTA (or absence of calcium) and antibodies which react only in the presence of antibiotic preservatives such as chloramphenicol. No single antibody detection method will detect all red cell antibodies; for instance MN and Duffy system antibodies cannot be detected using enzyme techniques and polybrene methods may miss Kell system antibodies. Generally, the more ingredients and variables there are in a test system, the more likelihood there is of false results.

Serum versus plasma for antibody detection

Traditionally, serum has been used in blood group serology for the detection of red cell antibodies. Clotted samples are simple to collect and a possible variable (the anticoagulant) is avoided. With the introduction of fully automated blood grouping systems, with probes that aspirate both plasma and cells, it has become necessary to use anticoagulated samples as the probes cannot aspirate cells from clotted samples. Anticoagulated plasma has been shown to be acceptable for the detection of IgG antibodies. However, if the anticoagulant acts by chelating calcium to prevent coagulation (e.g. EDTA or citrate), then the detection of complement fixed by clinically significant antibodies is not possible. This is particularly a problem with clinically significant complement fixing IgM antibodies, as they will not otherwise be detected in the AGT with modern polyspecific AHG (anti-IgG + anti-C3d). Additionally, antibody mediated haemolysis of red cells in screening or compatibility tests usually indicates a potentially very dangerous red cell antibody. This haemolysis will not be detected if EDTA plasma is used. In the author's laboratory the detection of clinically significant complement fixing antibodies is considered to be desirable and so an anticoagulant which is less likely to interfere with complement fixing (e.g. heparin) is favoured over EDTA or citrate.

Use of controls

Positive and negative controls are essential to show that test systems are working correctly. Controls should be processed under the same conditions as the tests. General guidance for the use of controls in blood group serology is given below.

Typing serum controls

- **Positive control.** The typing serum should be tested against a cell expressing a heterozygous or weak expression of the appropriate antigen.
- **Negative control.** The typing serum should be tested against a cell that is negative for the appropriate antigen.

Patient controls

- **Red cells.** When typing patient red cells, a negative control should be included of patient red cells reacted with patient's serum (auto-control) or reacted with an inert reagent control. This reagent control is essentially the inert diluent used for the typing serum. A positive reaction in this control (probably due to autoagglutination or polyagglutination) invalidates any positive test results.
- **Serum/plasma.** When ABO grouping a patient, a negative control of patient's serum with group O cells should be included. A positive result in this control indicates the presence of cold agglutinins other than anti-A or anti-B, and invalidates the test results.
- **Auto-control.** When performing cross-matching tests or antibody identifications, a control of patient red cells with patient serum should be included. A negative result in this control indicates that any positive test result must be due to alloantibody. A positive auto-control indicates that a positive test result may be due to an autoantibody or autoantibody + alloantibody. In this case further testing would be required to identify the problem.

Compatibility testing

This refers to all the procedures utilized in the selection and testing of a donor unit for transfusion to a patient. In this section just those procedures relevant to this chapter will be highlighted.

ABO and Rh D typing of donors and patients is best performed using robust, direct agglutination techniques in normal saline. Usually monoclonal typing reagents are used in tubes, microplates or microtubes. Typically, equal volumes of serum/plasma and a 3% suspension of red cells in saline are used. The test may be performed manually or may be automated. Reading of results is usually macroscopic and may involve the use of photometers or image analysis systems.

Screening for clinically significant red cell antibodies (in patients) is best performed using an LIS or NIS antiglobulin technique (AGT) at 37°C. The ratio of serum to cells should be at least 70 : 1. In the LIS-AGT, equal volumes of serum and cells must be used to maintain low ionic conditions. The tests are usually performed in tubes or microtubes, or in microplates using solid phase techniques. The tests may be performed manually or may be automated. Reading of tube tests is usually microscopic. However, with less experienced workers, the tip and roll technique has been shown to give fewer false negative results than microscopic reading. This is because the removal and transfer of red cells from a tube to a microscope slide using a pipette can, in inexperienced hands, lead to disruption of agglutination. Reading of microtube and microplate tests may be macroscopic or involve the use of photometers or image analysis systems.

Cross-matching, which involves testing patient serum/plasma against donor red cells, usually comprises a direct agglutination test and an AGT at 37°C. The direct agglutination test is performed immediately prior to incubating for the AGT. Its purpose is to rapidly indicate the presence of avid, direct agglutinating (complete) antibodies, especially those of the ABO system. The AGT, which may be LIS- or NIS-AGT, will detect clinically significant antibodies in most blood group systems (including ABO). Cross-matching tests are usually carried out in tubes and read microscopically, or in microtubes and read macroscopically or with the aid of photometers or image analysis systems.

Antibody identification

A detailed review of the procedures for identifying blood group antibodies is beyond the scope of this introductory text. However, the principles outlined in this chapter should give the student sufficient background to appreciate the wide variety of techniques available for the resolution of red cell antibodies and their limitations.

Suggested further reading

BCSH Blood Transfusion Task Force (1996). Guidelines for pre-transfusion compatibility procedures in blood transfusion laboratories. *Transfusion Medicine*, 6, 273–283.

Knight, R.C. and Poole, G.D. (1995). Detection of red cell antibodies: current and future techniques. *British Journal of Biomedical Science*, 52(4), 297–305.

Knight, R.C. and De Silva, M. (1996). New technologies for red-cell serology. *Blood Reviews*, 10, 101–110.

Phillips, P.K., Voak, D., Whitton, C.M. *et al.* (1993). BCSH–NIBSC anti-D reference reagent for antiglobulin tests: the in-house assessment of red cell washing centrifuges and of operator variability in the detection of weak, macroscopic agglutination. *Transfusion Medicine*, 3, 143–148.

Reviron, M. *et al.* (1984). The zeta potential and haemagglutination with Rh antibodies. *Vox Sang*, 46, 211–216.

van Oss, V.J. (1994). Immunological and physiological nature of antigen–antibody interactions. In *Immunobiology of Transfusion Medicine* (ed. G. Garratty). New York: Marcel Dekker, Inc.

van Oss, C.J. and Absolom, D.R. (1983). Zeta potentials, van der Waals forces and haemagglutination. *Vox Sang*, 44, 183–190.

Self-assessment questions

1. Name three factors that affect the first stage of agglutination.
2. What are the most likely causes of a false negative antiglobulin test?
3. How does treatment of red cells with proteolytic enzymes help to bring about direct agglutination with IgG antibodies?
4. Name four of the bonds or forces involved in antibody binding.
5. Why are IgM antibodies generally more likely than IgG antibodies to bring about direct agglutination of red cells suspended in saline?

Key Concepts and Facts

Haemagglutination

- Haemagglutination occurs in two stages: binding of antibody to red cell antigen and the formation of intercellular bridges between adjacent red cells.

- Binding of antibody to red cell antigen is a reversible, thermodynamic reaction.

- Red cells will naturally aggregate in order to lose surface free energy.

- This aggregation is opposed by the repulsive forces derived from the electronegative nature of the red cell membrane.

- Red cells suspended in ionized solutions such as saline attract clouds of cations. The electrical potentials related to the electronegative red cell surface and electropositive cation cloud appear as the zeta potential at the outer limit (slipping plane) of the cation cloud.

- The value of the zeta potential determines how closely red cells may approach one another. Typically this is 20 nm for red cells suspended in normal saline.

- IgM molecules can directly agglutinate saline-suspended red cells as they are large enough to bridge the gap between the red cells.

- IgG molecules are too small to bring about direct agglutination in saline. They may be detected by reducing the electrical charge surrounding the red cells, thus allowing the closer approach of the red cells, or indirectly by the addition of anti-IgG antibodies (the antiglobulin test).

Methods

- No single method will detect all clinically significant red cell antibodies.

- All enhancement methods and additives have the associated problem of causing false positive or negative reactions.

- The use of appropriate positive and negative controls is essential when antigen typing red cells or detecting red cell antibodies.

- Haemagglutination reactions may be visualized macroscopically, microscopically or with the aid of photometers or image analysis systems.

- Scoring of the agglutination reaction strengths can give valuable information.

Chapter 10
Adverse effects of blood transfusion

Learning objectives

After studying this chapter you should confidently be able to:

Describe the importance of donor selection.

List the tests performed on donor blood prior to release from the blood centre.

List the tests performed at the hospital transfusion laboratory prior to transfusion.

Describe the adverse effects due to red cell, platelet and plasma transfusions.

Describe the laboratory investigation of an alleged red cell transfusion reaction.

Outline the methods available to minimize the adverse effects of blood transfusion.

'Donating blood can be compared to sending a loaded gun to an unsuspecting or unprepared person. Like the loaded gun, there is a safety lever or button governing blood transfusion. But how many persons have died from gunshot wounds as the result of believing the lever was on "safe"?'

US Government report

Some definitions of terms used in this chapter are given below.

- **Blood component:** A term used to describe therapeutic material from a single donor. This includes red cells, platelet concentrates and fresh frozen plasma (FFP).

- **Plasma fraction:** A term used to describe therapeutic material derived from partially purified pools of donor plasma. This includes human albumin solution, coagulation factor concentrates and immunoglobulin preparations.

- **Blood product:** A term used to describe any therapeutic material prepared from human blood.

The transfusion of the correct blood product, to the correct patient, at the correct time, can make an important contribution to a patient's well-being or recovery, and may even be life-saving. However, every transfusion also carries a risk to the patient and may adversely affect the patient's well-being or recovery and may even be life-threatening.

When prescribing a blood transfusion or treatment with a human blood product, the clinician must balance the potential benefits to the patient with the potential risks.

The responsibilities of the transfusion scientist in the transfusion process are evident at every stage in the chain from production to supply. They are intimately involved in testing, treating, storing, issuing and investigating adverse reactions. It is vitally important, therefore, that they appreciate and understand the risks of transfusion and how they may be eliminated or minimized.

This chapter will look at the areas listed below.

- **General precautions:** donor selection and testing; blood product

The list below gives examples of criteria used in the selection of blood donors.

Blood will not be collected from potential donors who:

- Have a haemoglobin level of less than $135\,g\,l^{-1}$ for males and $125\,g\,l^{-1}$ for females.

- Have had a sore throat, cold or cough or any other infection in the last 7 days.

- Are currently taking painkillers.

- Have taken antibiotics, antihistamines or antidepressants in the last 7 days.

- Have had a local anaesthetic for dental treatment within the last 2 days.

- Have had a general anaesthetic for dental treatment within the last month.

- Are currently receiving medical treatment or attending a hospital for investigations.

- Have had a major operation within the last 6 months or a minor operation within the last month.

- Have had a child or a miscarriage within the last 12 months.

- Have recently had chickenpox, shingles, cold sores, measles, mumps or rubella, unless it is more than 3 weeks since they recovered.

- Know they are infected with HIV or have AIDS.

- Have injected themselves with drugs at any time since 1977.

- Have had sex since 1977 with men or women living in Africa.

- Are prostitutes.

collection, processing and storage; pre-transfusion testing; monitoring and reporting.

- **The adverse effects of transfusion** due to: disease transmission; red cells; white cells; platelets; plasma; other factors; and ways of minimizing the risks.

- **The investigation of an alleged red cell transfusion reaction**: the samples and information required; the tests to perform.

General precautions

The safety of all transfusions involves several elements relating to the donor, the blood sample and the patient. These are as follows:

- Selection of the donor.
- Testing of the donor.
- Blood product collection or manufacture.
- Blood product storage and transport.
- Collection of blood sample from the correct patient.
- Pre-transfusion testing of the patient's sample.
- Selection of appropriate blood product for the patient.
- Pre-transfusion treatment of the blood product where appropriate.
- Accurately identifying the patient prior to transfusion.
- Monitoring of the transfusion.
- Reporting of any adverse events.

Donor selection

The process of donor selection is designed to protect both the donor and the recipient. In the UK a donor must be a healthy person between the age of 17 and 70 years. They receive no payment for their donation. Donors either complete a questionnaire or are interviewed to identify those who could be harmed by donating and those whose donations could harm patients. Typical criteria used in the selection process are shown in the adjacent sidebox.

The emphasis is on identifying donors who carry a high risk for disease transmission, have a transmissible disorder, e.g. an allergy, or are taking medication which may affect the patient or the component being prepared, e.g. taking aspirin will adversely affect the quality of any platelet component produced. The system relies on the honesty of the donor, but as the intention of the overwhelming majority of donors is to help others, the system works well.

Donor testing

In the UK all blood donations are subjected to mandatory tests for hepatitis B virus (HBV), hepatitis C virus (HCV), human immuno-deficiency virus (HIV 1 and 2) and syphilis. Selected donations may also be tested for cytomegalovirus (CMV), for components to be transfused to neonates or immunocompromised patients. Blood donations are only released for issue to hospitals or fractionation centres for further processing if the results of these tests are negative.

All transfusion centres in the UK conduct microbiological surveillance of the donation, collection and processing procedures by taking appropriate samples for culture of micro-organisms from the donor, the storage and the laboratory environments and equipment used.

Blood donors have their ABO and Rhesus D types established at each donation. These results are compared with the results of previous tests (if any) held on a computer database. Blood is only released for issue if there is agreement between the current and historical results. The donor is also screened for atypical, clinically significant red cell antibodies. The blood is withheld if the results are positive.

Collection and storage

The blood donation must be collected as aseptically as possible, although total sterility is never achievable. The skin at the site of the venepuncture is cleansed with antiseptic, but bacteria below the surface of the skin may enter the venepuncture needle as may airborne bacteria. It is also quite possible for the donor to have an asymptomatic bacteraemia at the time of donation and bacteria in the circulation of the donor will enter the donation. Some of these bacteria will be destroyed by the activity of white blood cells in the donation, and surviving bacteria will have their proliferation curtailed by storage at 4–6°C. There are, however, some bacteria which are capable of growth even at low temperatures, e.g. *Pseudomonas fluorescens* and *Yersinia enterocolitica*. The risk of bacterial proliferation increases if the blood bag is allowed to warm to ambient temperature. For this reason transfusion must commence within 30 minutes of removal of the blood pack from the refrigerator, and be completed within 5 hours (for red cells). In addition, if the blood pack is removed from the refrigerator for further testing, processing or transportation, it must be returned to the correct storage temperature within 30 minutes to minimize the chance of bacterial proliferation within the pack. If the pack is allowed to warm for sufficient time for the bacteria to enter a logarithmic growth phase, then the bacterial load may have been increased by a factor of hundreds if not thousands. This situation will be exacerbated every time the blood pack is allowed to warm.

- Are men who have had sex with another man at any time since 1977.

- Are sexual partners of haemophiliacs.

Several disease-related tests are performed on blood donors in the UK, some mandatory and others optional.

The **mandatory tests** are for:

- HBV by testing for HBsAg (surface antigen).

- HCV by testing for antibodies.

- HIV 1 and 2 by testing for antibodies.

- Syphilis using the *Treponema pallidum* haemagglutination assay (TPHA), testing for antibodies.

The **optional tests** are for:

- CMV by testing for antibodies.

- Malaria by testing for antibodies.

Bacterial proliferation is an even greater problem with platelet components as these are stored at 22–24°C.

Bacteria may also enter components and plasma fractions during processing, and for this reason aseptic technique is again vital when handling and processing blood donations. At the blood transfusion centres processing usually takes place in specially designed donation packs with hermetically sealed transfer bags for separation of the various components, or by the attachment of transfer bags using sterile docking procedures.

At the hospital transfusion laboratory donor blood bags may have to be opened to allow removal of plasma or buffy coat, or to attach a leukocyte depletion filter. Again aseptic technique must be observed. Correct storage conditions after opening are essential to reduce the risk of bacterial proliferation, as are strict controls on the maximum time of storage following the opening of a blood bag. These times are usually 12 hours for red cells when stored between 4 and 6°C after opening and 6 hours for platelets stored between 22 and 24°C.

At the bedside the blood bags are opened to allow attachment of the blood-giving set. Again, aseptic technique is essential during this process.

Blood product selection, pre-treatment and pre-transfusion testing

The patient should be transfused with the most appropriate therapeutic product for their clinical condition. A wide range of blood products is available and it is important to be aware of the most appropriate product, its availability and the current guidelines for its use. (See Chapter 8 for more detailed information on the selection of appropriate therapeutic products.)

Pre-transfusion testing of the patient usually takes place at the hospital transfusion laboratory. The patient's ABO and Rhesus D type are established and the patient's serum/plasma is screened for atypical, clinically significant red cell antibodies.

In the case of red cell transfusions, the patient's serum/plasma is tested against the donor's red cells (cross-matched) by techniques designed to detect incompatibility due to ABO or other clinically significant red cell antibodies. Blood is usually only released for transfusion if these tests are negative.

Clerical errors may occur when taking the pre-transfusion blood sample from the patient, during laboratory testing or when transfusing blood. These errors are the most common causes of incompatible transfusions. A UK survey in 1994 indicated that of 111 incidents of patients receiving the wrong blood, 21% were due to the wrong patient's blood being sent to the laboratory, 5% were due to laboratory error and 74% were due to the ward or theatre transfusing blood to the wrong patient. One in 10 of all ABO incompatible transfusions resulted in the death of the patient.

Monitoring and reporting

Patients receiving a transfusion of any blood product must be monitored closely for the first 15 minutes of each unit transfused. In this way early clinical signs of acute reactions to incompatibilities or bacterial contamination can be detected. The patient should continue to be monitored regularly during and after the transfusion, to detect any signs of delayed reactions.

All used transfusion bags should be retained for a minimum of 24 hours after the blood transfusion is completed so that they are available for retesting in the event of any adverse reaction in the patient to the transfusion. If an adverse reaction is suspected during or after a transfusion, the hospital transfusion laboratory should be informed as soon as possible so that appropriate investigations can be instigated without delay (see below).

Suspected bacterial or viral infections caused by transfusion are reported as a matter of urgency to the local blood transfusion centre. Adverse reactions to plasma fractions, such as intravenous immunoglobulins, are reported to the Committee for the Safety of Medicines. Other serious adverse reactions resulting from the transfusion of blood components, e.g. acute haemolysis, delayed haemolysis and anaphylactic reactions, should be reported to the Serious Hazards of Transfusion (SHOT) group, using their confidential reporting system.

> The following is a summary with respect to reporting adverse reactions in the UK.
>
> - All adverse reactions should be reported to the hospital blood transfusion laboratory in the first instance.
>
> - Suspected bacterial or viral infections should be reported to the local blood transfusion centre.
>
> - Reactions to plasma fractions should be reported to the Committee for the Safety of Medicines.
>
> - Other serious adverse reactions should be reported to the Serious Hazards of Transfusion group.

Adverse effects

Disease transmission

The transfusion of blood products carries the very real risk of transmitting viral, bacterial or protozoal infections from the donor to the patient.

Viral infections most often reported in association with blood transfusion include human immunodeficiency virus (HIV), hepatitis B virus (HBV), hepatitis C virus (HCV), cytomegalovirus (CMV), hepatitis A virus (HAV), Epstein–Barr virus (EBV) and parvovirus B19. Testing donors for HIV, HBV and HCV is mandatory but donors in the 'window period' of an infection may not be detected. The 'window period' is that time between infection and seroconversion when a donor is infectious but is still seronegative with respect to the virus being tested for.

The risks may be minimized by:

- Careful selection of donors.
- Laboratory testing for HIV, HBV, HCV and CMV.
- Solvent/detergent treatment of plasma fractions to inactivate enveloped viruses.
- Heat and/or chemical treatment of plasma fractions.
- Leukocyte depletion of red cell and platelet components to reduce

What follows is a case history illustrating a delayed transfusion reaction.

An 85-year-old female (C.G.) was admitted to hospital on the 26 February for elective total hip replacement surgery. On admission she had a low haemoglobin (Hb) level of $85\,g\,l^{-1}$ and a raised mean cell volume (MCV) of 105 fl. A blood film examination indicated a possible folate deficiency. She was immediately started on folate and vitamin B12 treatment and transfused two units of red cells. Surgery was deferred.

At this time C.G. grouped as O Rh D positive with no clinically significant antibodies detected. The two units of red cells were compatible in the cross-match and were transfused uneventfully.

On 14 May the patient was readmitted. Her Hb was now $120\,g\,l^{-1}$ with an MCV of 103 fl. No clinically significant antibodies were detected in her serum and two units of cross-match compatible red cells were transfused uneventfully during surgery on 18 May.

Post-operatively on 21 May her Hb had fallen to $88\,g\,l^{-1}$, although there had been no significant post-operative blood loss. She complained of feeling generally unwell and had a slight fever, although there was no evidence of a post-operative infection. A sample was sent for cross-matching of red cells to correct the anaemia. The units of red cells cross-matched were found to be incompatible (gave positive results) in the indirect antiglobulin test and the auto-control (patient's red cells tested with patient's serum) was positive.

The patient's serum was shown to contain the Rh antibody anti-E. The direct antiglobulin test performed on the patient's red cell

the risk of CMV transmission as the virus is carried within white cells.

- The presence of antibodies to HAV and parvovirus B19 in plasma pools. Up to 60% of normal donors have antibodies to these viruses in their plasma.

Bacterial infections transmitted by blood transfusion can be rapidly fatal for the patient. As previously mentioned, bacteria may enter the blood supply at the time of collection or during subsequent processing. Some bacteria, e.g. *Yersinia enterocolitica*, are capable of proliferating even during refrigerated storage of blood.

The risks may be minimized by:

- Careful selection of donors.
- Laboratory testing in the case of *Treponema pallidum* (which causes syphilis).
- Microbiological surveillance of the donor, storage and testing environments.
- Strict adherence to storage temperatures.
- Not allowing blood to be out of a refrigerator for more than 30 minutes prior to transfusion.
- Limiting storage times after components have been opened for processing.
- Use of aseptic techniques during processing.

Protozoal infections most often reported in connection with blood transfusion include malaria, babesiosis, toxoplasmosis and filariasis. No laboratory testing procedures for these organisms are routinely conducted in the UK. The risks of transmission are minimized by careful donor selection and the rejection of donors who have recently visited areas where any of these infections are endemic.

Adverse reactions due to the transfusion of red cells

The most serious reaction to a red cell transfusion is that of **acute intravascular haemolysis** of the donor red cells by haemolytic red cell antibodies in the patient. These are usually ABO antibodies. The destruction of red cells, activation of complement and release of haemoglobin leads rapidly to disseminated intravascular coagulation, acute renal failure and shock, and is fatal in at least 10% of cases. The majority of ABO-incompatible transfusions occur due to clerical errors in the identification of the patient at the time of sampling, collection of blood from the laboratory or at the time of transfusion.

The risk may be minimized by:

- Accurate blood grouping and labelling of donor units.
- Accurate blood grouping of patients.
- Pre-transfusion testing to detect ABO or other haemolytic antibodies.
- Accurate identification of the patient at the time of sampling.
- Accurate identification of the patient and donor unit at the time of collection from the laboratory.
- Accurate identification of the patient prior to transfusion.

Delayed (extravascular) haemolysis of transfused red cells may be caused by antibodies to several different blood group systems (see Chapter 6). The patient's haemoglobin level will fall as the transfused donor red cells are destroyed and the patient may suffer from a fever and general malaise. Future transfusions must be with red cells which have been typed and shown to be negative with respect to the patient's antibody.

The risk may be minimized by:

- Pre-transfusion screening of the patient's serum/plasma for clinically significant red cell antibodies.
- Cross-matching the patient's serum/plasma against the donor red cells.

Alloimmunization to many different red cell antigens will occur at every transfusion, as the donor red cells will normally only be matched with the patient's ABO and Rh D type. After a patient has received a transfusion of red cells any further transfusions should be preceded by antibody screening and cross-matching with a sample taken at least 3 days after the last transfusion. This is to allow sufficient time for any newly formed antibodies to appear in the serum/plasma. If a patient does develop red cell antibodies this could lead to difficulties in supplying blood in the future or to haemolytic disease of the newborn in subsequent pregnancies.

The risk may be minimized by:

- Only transfusing red cells when absolutely necessary.
- Treatment with iron rather than red cells to correct iron deficiency anaemia.
- The use of recombinant erythropoietin to stimulate the patient's own red cell production.

Iron overload is a particular risk with patients who receive regular red cell transfusions over many months or years. The accumulation of iron from transfused red cells can lead to widespread tissue damage and interference with hepatic function. The risk may be minimized by treating the patient with chelation therapy, e.g. desferrioxamine, to eliminate unwanted iron.

Figure 10.1 illustrates the adverse reaction risks associated with the transfusion of red cell products.

sample was positive with an IgG antibody shown to be coating the red cells. This antibody was eluted from the red cells and was identified as anti-E.

Two units of O Rh D positive, E negative red cells were cross-matched and found to be compatible. C.G. was transfused both units uneventfully on 27 May. Her Hb rose to $122\,\text{g}\,\text{l}^{-1}$ and remained steady throughout the rest of her hospital stay.

The explanation for the above case history is as follows. The patient had been immunized by the transfusion of E positive red cells to correct the pre-operative anaemia on 4 March. The anti-E produced as a result of this immunization was too weak to be detected when red cells were cross-matched for the surgery on 18 May. One or both of the units transfused during surgery on 18 May was E positive. The patient did not react immediately to this fresh immunization but had a delayed reaction (secondary antibody response) 3 days later, which caused a fall in her Hb level as the transfused red cells were destroyed by her antibody. The positive direct antiglobulin test was detecting the patient's antibody bound to transfused donor red cells still in her circulation. The transfusion of red cells which were negative with respect to her anti-E antibody successfully corrected her anaemia.

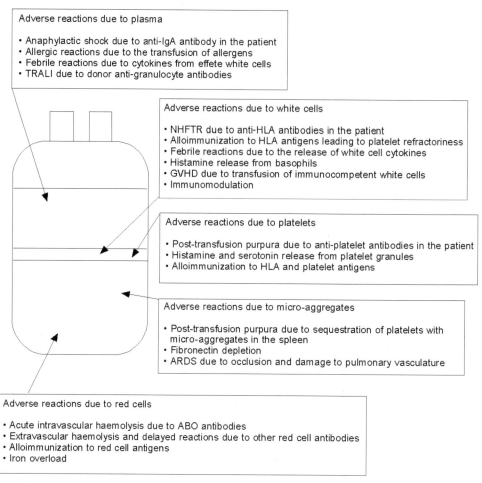

Adverse reactions due to plasma

- Anaphylactic shock due to anti-IgA antibody in the patient
- Allergic reactions due to the transfusion of allergens
- Febrile reactions due to cytokines from effete white cells
- TRALI due to donor anti-granulocyte antibodies

Adverse reactions due to white cells

- NHFTR due to anti-HLA antibodies in the patient
- Alloimmunization to HLA antigens leading to platelet refractoriness
- Febrile reactions due to the release of white cell cytokines
- Histamine release from basophils
- GVHD due to transfusion of immunocompetent white cells
- Immunomodulation

Adverse reactions due to platelets

- Post-transfusion purpura due to anti-platelet antibodies in the patient
- Histamine and serotonin release from platelet granules
- Alloimmunization to HLA and platelet antigens

Adverse reactions due to micro-aggregates

- Post-transfusion purpura due to sequestration of platelets with micro-aggregates in the spleen
- Fibronectin depletion
- ARDS due to occlusion and damage to pulmonary vasculature

Adverse reactions due to red cells

- Acute intravascular haemolysis due to ABO antibodies
- Extravascular haemolysis and delayed reactions due to other red cell antibodies
- Alloimmunization to red cell antigens
- Iron overload

Figure 10.1   *Adverse reaction risks with the transfusion of red cell products (see text for details)*

Adverse reactions due to the transfusion of white cells

Non-haemolytic febrile transfusion reactions (NHFTRs) occur in as many as 1% of all transfusions and in up to 45% of patients receiving multiple transfusions. The patient may experience flushing, pyrexia, rigors and hypotension. The reactions are caused by anti-white cell antibodies in the patient reacting with donor white cells to activate complement, causing the release of pyrogens and vasoactive amines. Similar reactions can occur due to the **release of cytokines** from damaged donor white cells. Likewise, **histamine** released from effete donor basophils may cause urticarial reactions or bronchospasm and hypotension in the patient. These risks may be minimized by removing the donor white cells (leuko-depletion) from any red cell or platelet components prior to transfusion.

Post-transfusion purpura (PTP) may occur due to the sequestration of platelets into the spleen in association with transfused micro-aggregates. These micro-aggregates occur in all donations of red cells and comprise an aggregate of fibrin, donor white cells and platelets. The number and size of these aggregates increase with the length of storage of the donated blood. Micro-aggregates have also been implicated in **reducing fibronectin levels** in transfused patients. The risk may be minimized by removal of micro-aggregates by filtration immediately prior to transfusion, particularly for patients receiving massive transfusions.

Adult respiratory distress syndrome (ARDS) may be caused by occlusion of the pulmonary vasculature by transfused micro-aggregates. This can lead to the release of free oxygen radicals and lysosomal enzymes and complement activation with conse-quent damage to the lungs. The risk may be minimized by removal of micro-aggregates by filtration immediately prior to transfusion, particularly for patients receiving massive transfusions.

Graft versus host disease (GVHD) is an often fatal condition brought about by the transfusion of immunocompetent white cells to an immunocompromised patient. The donor white cells prolif-erate in the host (patient) and reject a variety of host tissues (see Chapter 11). The risk may be minimized by irradiating red cell and platelet components prior to transfusion to kill the donor white cells.

Alloimmunization to many different white cell antigens will occur at every transfusion. This may lead to the production of anti-HLA antibodies (see Chapter 11), which are not only implicated in the NHFTRs mentioned previously but may cause the patient to become **refractory to platelet transfusions.** That is to say, the anti-HLA antibodies can destroy transfused platelets so that the patient does not get the expected benefit from platelet transfusions. In this case, the patient would have to be transfused with platelets from an HLA-matched donor. Finding HLA-matched donors can be very difficult, time-consuming and expensive. The risk may be minimized by removing the donor white cells (leuko-depletion) from any red cell or platelet components prior to transfusion. This is especially important for patients who are receiving long-term red cell or platelet transfusion support.

Immunomodulation following transfusion refers to a temporary impairment of the patient's immune system. This may manifest itself in the form of an increased chance of tumour recurrence following surgery for tumour removal, or an increased incidence of post-operative infections, in patients receiving blood transfusions. The precise mechanism of this effect is unknown, but the most popular theories attribute the effect to the transfusion of white cells. The risk may be minimized by removing the donor white cells from any red cell or platelet components prior to transfusion.

Adverse reactions due to the transfusion of platelets

Alloimmunization to many different platelet antigens will occur at every transfusion. This may lead to the production of anti-platelet antibodies. Platelet components may be contaminated with red cells and white cells, which may stimulate the patient to produce red cell or anti-HLA antibodies. The anti-HLA antibodies may cause the patient to become **refractory to platelet transfusions** as described previously. **Post-transfusion purpura** (PTP) caused by anti-platelet antibodies present in the patient may cause a life-threatening thrombocytopenia.

The risk may be minimized by:

- The selection of platelets from matched donors once the anti-platelet antibody has been identified.
- Selecting platelets from Rh D negative donors for transfusion to Rh D females of childbearing age, to prevent the patient being immunized to produce anti-D.
- Administration of prophylactic anti-D to any Rh D negative female of childbearing age who has received platelets from an Rh D positive donor.
- Removing the donor white cells from platelet components prior to transfusion to avoid the patient being stimulated to produce anti-HLA antibodies.

Histamine and serotonin release from damaged donor platelets can cause urticaria, bronchospasm and hypotension. There is no specific measure available to minimize this risk, but fortunately the symptoms are usually not severe and may be treated with antihistamines.

Acute haemolysis of patient red cells by donor ABO antibodies present in the supernatant plasma of the platelet component is a potential hazard, but fortunately this is a rare occurrence. The risk may be minimized by selecting platelets from ABO-compatible donors.

Figure 10.2 illustrates the adverse reaction risks associated with the transfusion of platelet products.

Adverse reactions due to the transfusion of plasma

Anaphylactic reactions are extremely rare but have a high mortality rate. They are usually caused by a reaction between anti-IgA in the patient's serum and the IgA contained in the transfused plasma.

The risk may be minimized by:

- The use of products from IgA-deficient donors for future transfusions.

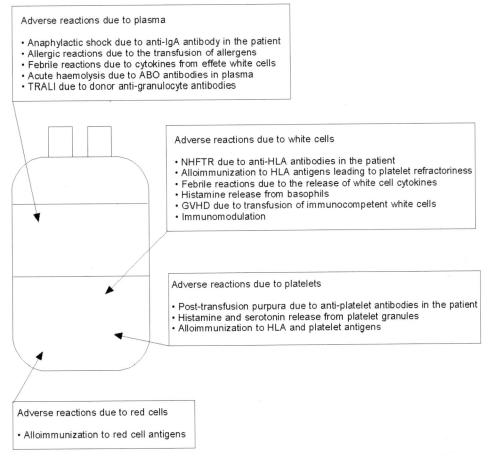

Adverse reactions due to plasma

• Anaphylactic shock due to anti-IgA antibody in the patient
• Allergic reactions due to the transfusion of allergens
• Febrile reactions due to cytokines from effete white cells
• Acute haemolysis due to ABO antibodies in plasma
• TRALI due to donor anti-granulocyte antibodies

Adverse reactions due to white cells

• NHFTR due to anti-HLA antibodies in the patient
• Alloimmunization to HLA antigens leading to platelet refractoriness
• Febrile reactions due to the release of white cell cytokines
• Histamine release from basophils
• GVHD due to transfusion of immunocompetent white cells
• Immunomodulation

Adverse reactions due to platelets

• Post-transfusion purpura due to anti-platelet antibodies in the patient
• Histamine and serotonin release from platelet granules
• Alloimmunization to HLA and platelet antigens

Adverse reactions due to red cells

• Alloimmunization to red cell antigens

Figure 10.2 *Adverse reaction risks with the transfusion of platelet products (see text for details)*

• Transfusing red cells and platelet components that have been washed free of plasma.

Transfusion-related acute lung injury (TRALI) is most usually caused by anti-granulocyte antibodies in the donor plasma reacting with the patient's granulocytes. Complement is activated and granulocyte breakdown occurs primarily in the pulmonary vasculature, leading to non-cardiogenic pulmonary oedema and infiltration of the lower lung. The condition is potentially fatal. The risk may be minimized by identifying donors who have been implicated in cases of TRALI and removing them from the regular donor panels.

Allergic reactions to plasma (FFP or platelet or red cell supernatant) are very common and are usually caused by the reaction between an allergen in the transfused plasma and patient antibody or, more unusually, by an allergy passively acquired from the donor. **Febrile reactions** may also occur due to the presence of

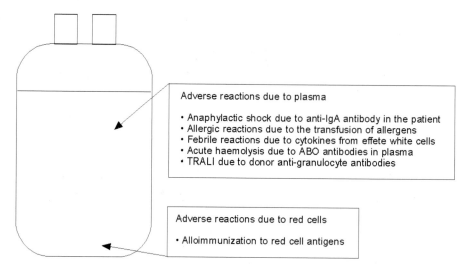

Adverse reactions due to plasma

- Anaphylactic shock due to anti-IgA antibody in the patient
- Allergic reactions due to the transfusion of allergens
- Febrile reactions due to cytokines from effete white cells
- Acute haemolysis due to ABO antibodies in plasma
- TRALI due to donor anti-granulocyte antibodies

Adverse reactions due to red cells

- Alloimmunization to red cell antigens

Figure 10.3   *Adverse reaction risks with the transfusion of plasma products (see text for details)*

cytokines that have been released into the plasma from damaged donor white cells.

The risk may be minimized by:

- Careful selection of donors to eliminate those with known allergies.
- Removing the donor white cells from any red cell or platelet components (preferably pre-storage).

Alloimmunization to red cell antigens may occur due to the small amounts of red cell stroma found in standard FFP preparations. **Acute haemolysis** of patient red cells by donor ABO antibodies present in FFP may also occur.

The risks may be minimized by:

- Selecting FFP from Rh D negative donors for transfusion to Rh D negative females of childbearing age, to prevent the patient being immunized to produce anti-D.
- Administration of prophylactic anti-D to any Rh D negative female of childbearing age who has received FFP from an Rh D positive donor.
- Selection of FFP from ABO-compatible donors.

Figure 10.3 illustrates the adverse reaction risks associated with the transfusion of plasma products.

Adverse reactions due to other causes

Circulatory overload, **air embolism** and **thrombophlebitis** at the infusion site are conditions which may complicate all intravenous infusions. The risk of them occurring is minimized by good clinical practice.

Toxicity caused by the transfusion of citrate in the anticoagulant or potassium that has leaked from red cells may be a problem for patients receiving massive transfusions in a short space of time. Toxicity caused by PVC or phthalate plasticizers which dissolve from the blood pack into the donor blood are a theoretical rather than a practical risk with modern blood packs.

Unusual reactions include reports of patients who developed **acute hypersensitivity reactions** during transfusion. These reactions were due to the patients having an IgE antibody which acted against residual ethylene oxide contained in the blood-giving sets. The ethylene oxide had been used to sterilize the sets. Patients have also been reported who developed an **urticarial rash** due to a sensitivity to the nickel coating on the transfusion needle.

A much more serious risk is that of **hypothermia** and **cardiac arrest** brought on by the rapid transfusion of large volumes of cold blood. This risk may be minimized by the use of a blood warmer at the time of transfusion.

Investigation of an alleged reaction to a red cell transfusion

The most common adverse reactions are not due to red cell antibodies but are febrile or urticarial reactions due to white cell antibodies, cytokines or allergens.

These types of reaction also account for most of the immediate (or during transfusion) reactions and are usually not life-threatening, although they may be very uncomfortable and disconcerting for the patient. Immediate reactions caused by bacterial contamination or red cell incompatibility (usually ABO) are much rarer occurrences but can be rapidly fatal. A more common occurrence when red cell antibodies are present is the delayed transfusion reaction, which may occur 3–14 days post-transfusion. It may only be detected because of a falling haemoglobin level due to destruction of transfused red cells, spherocytes in a blood smear, a positive direct antiglobulin test or positive auto-control in a subsequent cross-match (see Chapter 9). A delayed transfusion reaction is caused by a delayed secondary antibody response in the patient to the transfused red cells. Pre-transfusion the antibody is at such a low level as to be not detectable. Reactions which occur during a transfusion should be reported to the hospital transfusion laboratory, preferably as soon as possible after they occur and after the patient has been stabilized. The transfusion laboratory must then obtain the following information and blood samples in order to investigate the reaction to the transfusion:

- A relevant history from the patient, which should include information concerning any previous transfusions, previous reac-

Blood products are subjected to various pre-treatment regimes to minimize the risks of an adverse reaction, as outlined below.

Removal of white cells (**leukocyte depletion**) from red cell and platelet components prior to transfusion reduces the risk of an adverse reaction in several ways.

Pre-storage leukocyte depletion refers to the removal of leukocytes from the donation, usually by filtration, 24–72 hours **after collection**. This process can reduce the risk of:

- Immunization to HLA antigens carried on the white cells.

- Febrile reactions caused by a patient's anti-HLA antibodies reacting with donor white cells.

- CMV transmission, as the virus is carried in white cells.

- Impairment of the patient's immune system (immunomodulation).

- Febrile reactions caused by cytokines released into the donor plasma from effete donor white cells.

- Reactions caused by the release of histamine into the donor plasma from effete donor basophils.

Post-storage leukocyte depletion refers to the removal of leukocytes from red cell or platelet components, usually by filtration, immediately **prior to transfusion**, either in the laboratory or at the bedside. This process can reduce the risk of:

- Immunization to HLA antigens carried on the white cells.

- Febrile reactions caused by a patient's anti-HLA antibodies reacting with donor white cells.

- CMV transmission, as the virus is carried in white cells.

- Impairment of the patient's immune system (immunomodulation).

The 1993 consensus conference of the Royal College of Physicians of Edinburgh recommended a level of less than 5×10^6 residual white cells per red cell unit or platelet dose for effective leukocyte depletion in most cases. Modern leukocyte depletion filters are capable of achieving this level by removing more than 99.9% of leukocytes from a blood donation.

Irradiation of red cell or platelet components with gamma radiation removes the risk of graft versus host disease (GVHD) by inactivating immunocompetent donor leukocytes. The British Committee for Standards in Haematology (1996) recommends that each component bag should receive a dose of gamma radiation of not less than 25 Gy and not more than 50 Gy.

Virus inactivation of donor plasma to reduce the risk of disease transmission may be achieved in several ways. For example, plasma fractions and plasma pools may be treated with heat or with a combination of solvent and detergent. Fresh frozen plasma may be treated with methylene blue which irreversibly denatures viruses on exposure to light.

tions, any history of HDNB, previous pregnancies, and drugs and medication currently being taken.

- A pre-transfusion serum/plasma sample.
- A post-transfusion serum/plasma sample.
- A post-transfusion DAT sample.
- A post-transfusion urine sample.
- The remains of any used blood packs.
- The remains of the offending unit of blood with the blood-giving set still *in situ*. The blood in the pack will be examined for bacterial contamination. Leaving the set still attached to the blood pack prevents any new bacterial contamination of the blood.
- Any untransfused units of blood.

The tests that should be performed are shown in Table 10.1. Sometimes, the pre-transfusion samples and donor units may no longer be available. In this case the post-transfusion samples should be tested as shown in Table 10.2. Further, more elaborate, tests may need to be performed in addition to those shown in Tables

Table 10.1   *Tests required for the investigation of an alleged reaction to a red cell transfusion*

Sample	Tests
Pre-transfusion blood sample from the patient	Repeat ABO and Rh group Repeat antibody screen Identify any antibodies detected Repeat cross-match of all units of blood
Post-transfusion blood sample from the patient	ABO and Rh group Antibody screen Identify any antibodies detected DAT Cross-match of all units of blood
Donor blood units	Check for correct labelling of units of blood Check ABO and Rh group Antigen type for any antibodies found in pre- or post-transfusion samples
Post-transfusion urine sample from the patient	Examine for signs of haemolysis
The offending unit of blood	Send for microbiological testing (this usually involves testing samples from the pack, side-tube and giving set)

Table 10.2 *Tests required for the investigation of an alleged reaction to a red cell transfusion when only the post-transfusion sample is available*

Sample	Tests
Post-transfusion blood sample from the patient	ABO and Rh group Antibody screen DAT Identify any antibodies found Blood smear to check for spherocytes

10.1 and 10.2. However, such test procedures are beyond the scope of this introductory text.

Summary

After reading this chapter the student may be forgiven for wondering how any patient ever survives a blood transfusion. The dangers and complications of transfusion are myriad but in practice the vast majority of transfusions are uneventful. This is thanks, in large part, to the knowledge and skills of the staff of the blood transfusion centres, fractionation centres and hospital blood transfusion laboratories, and of course to the commitment and honesty of the blood donors.

Techniques available to detect clinically significant antibodies, to prepare safe and effective blood products, to minimize disease transmission and reduce the other risks associated with blood transfusion are now very sophisticated. However, the transfusion community must not become complacent. There are still risks which need to be investigated and minimized, such as immunomodulation and the risk of virus transmission in red cell and platelet components. Adverse reactions are under-reported by nursing and clinical staff, so the real frequency of occurrence of many types of adverse reactions is still unknown.

Suggested further reading

Blood Transfusion Services of the United Kingdom (1996). *Handbook of Transfusion Medicine* (ed. D.B.L. McClelland). London: HMSO.

UKBTS/NIBSC Liaison Group (1996). *Guidelines for the Blood Transfusion Services in the United Kingdom*. Leeds: National Blood Service.

Self-assessment questions

1. In the UK, mandatory testing of blood donations involves testing for which transmissible diseases?
2. What is the most common cause of an incompatible red cell transfusion?
3. What are the most common types of transfusion reaction?
4. To whom should adverse transfusion reactions be reported?
5. How may the risk of graft versus host disease be minimized?
6. Apart from alloimmunization and reactions to red cell antibodies, what is the other major danger of repeated red cell transfusions?
7. What are the two mechanisms by which post-transfusion purpura may occur in a patient?
8. How may the risk of viral transmission from transfusion be minimized?
9. Following an alleged red cell transfusion reaction, what tests should be performed on the patient's post-transfusion samples?

Key Concepts and Facts

Possible Adverse Effects

- The transfusion of the correct blood product to the correct patient at the correct time can be life-saving.

- However, the complications and possible adverse outcomes of blood transfusion can be life-threatening.

- Blood transfusion may transmit bacterial, protozoal or viral infections to the patient.

- Various adverse reactions may be caused by the transfusion of red cells, white cells, platelets or plasma.

How the Risks may be Minimized:

- Careful selection of donors to eliminate those whose donations may harm patients.

- Donor testing for ABO, Rh D type and clinically significant red cell antibodies.

- Donor testing for HBV, HCV, HIV, syphilis and, in some cases, CMV.

- Applying procedures to minimize bacterial contamination during blood collection, processing, storage and transport.

- Correct identification of the patient when taking samples and administering transfusions.

- Patient pre-transfusion testing for ABO, Rh D type and clinically significant red cell antibodies.

- Cross-matching of patient serum with donor red cells.

- Careful monitoring of the patient during the transfusion.

- Prompt reporting and investigation of adverse reactions.

- Pre-transfusion filtering of blood components to remove white cells.

- Pre-transfusion irradiation of blood components to inactivate donor white cells.

- Pre-transfusion treatment of plasma fractions to inactivate viruses.

Chapter 11
Transplantation

Learning objectives

After studying this chapter you should confidently be able to:

Discuss the classification of different grafts based on genetic relationships between donor and recipient.

Discuss the immunological causes of graft rejection and graft versus host disease.

Discuss the structure of major histocompatibility antigens and their role in graft rejection.

Describe the HLA system and discuss its polymorphic nature.

Outline methods for tissue typing.

Outline the reasons for carrying out a stem cell transplant.

Discuss the different sources of stem cells for transplantation.

Tissue transplantation involves the transfer of tissues or organs either within one individual or between two individuals. Transplants of tissues from one human to another have been carried out with a degree of success since Joseph Murray performed the first successful kidney transplant in 1954 (see Table 11.1). In

Table 11.1 *Some landmarks in clinical transplantation*

Year	Landmark
1943	Medawar establishes that the immune system causes graft rejection
1954	First successful human kidney transplant
1958	Discovery of HLA antigens
1967	First human heart transplant
1968	First successful human bone marrow transplant
1968	First human liver transplants
1977	Use of autologous bone marrow reported
1986	First peripheral blood stem cell transplant
1987	First umbilical cord stem cell transplant

Table 11.2 *Tissue and organ transplants*

Tissue transplanted	Examples of clinical condition
Skin	Plastic surgery, e.g. for treatment of burns
Cornea	Types of blindness
Kidney	End-stage renal failure
Heart	Coronary heart disease
Heart and lungs	Cystic fibrosis
Pancreas	Insulin dependent diabetes mellitus
Liver	Cirrhosis
Bone marrow	Immune deficiency; in treatment of leukaemia
Bone	Orthopaedic surgery
Foetal brain cell	Parkinson's disease*
Foetal thymus	Immune deficiency*

* Currently experimental.

1967, Christiaan Barnard performed the first human heart transplant and in doing so opened up the field to intense media interest. Nowadays, kidney and heart transplants have become more frequent and the range of tissues transplanted is extensive (see Table 11.2). Although tissue transplants are becoming routine, the process is not without its difficulties, the most obvious one being that, if the graft comes from an individual who is not genetically identical to the recipient (as for example when a graft is carried out between identical twins – a rare event), then the immune system of the recipient is highly likely to destroy the transplanted tissues which are recognized as foreign or 'non-self'.

The most common types of grafts, which include kidney, heart, liver, lung, pancreas and corneal transplants, are those in which the aim is to replace a defective organ. Such grafts are invariably given to people who have a properly functioning immune system. In these cases, the person who receives the graft is likely to mount an immune response against the graft (if the graft is not antigenically identical to the tissues of the donor) unless immunosuppressive treatments are given. The success of these transplants has been due to advances on several fronts, including a greater understanding of the immune system, better immunosuppressive drugs, improved laboratory methods for matching donor and recipient, and even the advent of computer databases to 'match' a potential graft to a potential recipient (sometimes worldwide).

Transplants of bone marrow as well as thymus present particular problems not usually associated with other types of transplant, since these are usually given to treat an immunodeficiency – sometimes one that has been caused by clinical treatments. For example, bone marrow transplants may be given to individuals who have had highly toxic chemical or radiation treatments to destroy deposits of leukaemic cells in bone marrow. In such cases the recipient (or host) cannot reject the graft but the graft, which contains mature cells of the immune system (immunocompetent cells), can recognize the recipient as foreign and mount an attack on the cells of the recipient. Such an occurrence is called a **graft versus host reaction** and it causes **graft versus host disease (GVHD)** which can be fatal.

This chapter will look at the immunological basis of graft rejection and how this relates to bone marrow transplantation in particular. In addition, this chapter will discuss ways in which patients can be 'matched' to potential donors in such a way as to minimize the chances of rejection occurring.

Major histocompatibility antigens

Whether or not a graft is rejected depends on genetic differences between individuals, and the greater the genetic difference, the greater the chances of rejection. These genetic differences relate to the expression of cell surface proteins encoded by a region of the genome called the **major histocompatibility complex (MHC)**. The cell surface proteins encoded by the MHC are fundamentally important in the immune response because they 'present' foreign antigens to T lymphocytes (see Chapter 1). Class I MHC molecules present antigens to CD8+ cytotoxic T lymphocytes whereas Class II molecules present antigens to CD4+ helper T lymphocytes. It is differences between the MHC molecules on the cells of the graft and the cells of the host that stimulate graft rejection. It is, however, important to remember that MHC proteins are not present for the sole purpose of causing difficulties for transplant surgeons, even if they were discovered in that context.

Relationships between donor and recipient

The main factor which determines whether a graft will be rejected or accepted is the genetic disparity between the donor tissue and the recipient. The wider this disparity, then the more likely the graft is to be rejected. Table 11.3 shows how grafts are classified according to these genetic relationships. **Isografts** or **autografts** are often used in plastic surgery as, for example, when healthy skin is used to treat a badly burned area. When bone marrow from one individual is administered to the same individual this is most commonly called an **autologous** graft. Isografts or autografts are not rejected since they are obviously genetically identical to the recipient.

The most common type of clinical transplant is an **allograft**. These grafts are always likely to be rejected. Immunosuppressive drugs have to be used to prevent rejection occurring, even if there is a good match for MHC proteins. Syngeneic grafts are not relevant clinically. Xenogeneic grafts have been used as, for example, when a heart from a baboon has been implanted into a human. Transgenic grafts in humans are xenogeneic grafts from animals which have

The term **histocompatibility** refers to whether a tissue will be accepted or rejected by an individual. MHC molecules were first discovered as a result of investigations by scientists such as Snell and Gorer into the genetics of the rejection of transplanted tumours in mice. They discovered a genetic region containing a complex set of genes coding for 'histocompatibility antigens'. This genetic region is known as the H2 region and is the murine MHC.

Table 11.3 *Definitions of transplants*

Name	Alternative	Relationship between donor and recipient
Isograft	Autograft (autologous graft)	Tissue is transplanted from one part of an individual to another part of the same individual
Allograft	Allogeneic graft	Tissue is transplanted between two individuals of the same species
Syngeneic graft		Tissue is transplanted between two individuals of a highly inbred strain of animals
Xenogeneic graft	Heterograft	Tissue is transplanted between two individuals of different species
Transgenic graft		Tissue is transplanted between two individuals, usually of different species, where the donor has been genetically engineered to express some genes of the recipient

been genetically engineered to express human MHC antigens. Currently this work is experimental. Transgenic pigs have been developed to carry human antigens but there is currently much debate about the ethics of transplanting organs from such animals into humans. Transgenic transplantation is most unlikely to be useful in bone marrow transplantation where it is much more important to find histocompatible donors to prevent the development of GVHD. In order to understand the particular problems associated with bone marrow transplantation, it is first necessary to understand something about how the immune system actually destroys grafts.

What causes graft rejection?

The rejection of grafts is brought about by cells of the immune system. Rejection of organ transplants may take place within hours of the organ being attached to the blood supply of the recipient (**hyperacute rejection**). The more usual type of rejection takes place a few weeks after transplantation and is known as **acute rejection**. Sometimes there is a **chronic rejection** process, which takes place months or even years after a transplant. Different immunological mechanisms underlie these different responses.

Acute rejection

There is abundant evidence to show that acute rejection of grafts is brought about by a cell-mediated immune response and not by

The eminent immunologist Sir Peter Medawar was among the first to demonstrate that the rejection of an allograft was an immunological phenomenon. Using skin grafts in animals, he showed that a second graft was rejected more quickly than a first graft if the second graft was genetically identical to the first. This demonstrates both specificity and immunological memory, which are hallmarks of the specific immune response. In transplantation immunology, rejection of the first graft is called a **first set** response. The quicker rejection of the second graft is called a **second set** response. These terms are analogous to the terms more usually used in immunology, i.e. the primary and secondary responses (see Chapter 1).

The immune response is not directed against an entire MHC protein but merely against those regions which are different from the recipient's own MHC molecules. Transplantation scientists therefore tend to talk about MHC **antigens** rather than MHC proteins since it is the antigens that are the main focus of interest. It is only necessary to remember that the antigens are regions of the MHC molecules to which antibodies bind.

antibodies. For example, animals that have no T cells do not reject grafts. It can also be shown that grafts which are undergoing rejection become infiltrated with T lymphocytes and monocytes, a strong indication of cell-mediated immunity.

T lymphocytes (both CD4+ and CD8+) respond to the foreign histocompatibility antigens on the surface of the donated cells. The immune system produces cytotoxic T lymphocytes (CTL) directed against the foreign histocompatibility antigens on the grafted cells. CTL are capable of killing cells of the grafts directly or indirectly by releasing cytokines which attract and activate phagocytes, particularly monocytes and macrophages (see Chapter 1). In addition, sensitized CD4+ (helper) T lymphocytes respond by producing cytokines which activate a variety of non-specific cells to destroy the graft.

Hyperacute rejection

Although antibodies may be produced against transplanted tissue, they do not usually cause rejection unless these antibodies are already present when the tissue is grafted. These 'preformed' antibodies can cause a hyperacute rejection. Hyperacute rejection can be brought about if the recipient already has antibody to MHC antigens present on the graft.

Several types of patient may have preformed antibody to MHC proteins. These include:

- Women who have had a number of pregnancies (multiparous). Such women have been exposed to 'foreign' MHC antigens on the cells of the foetus and have become immunized to these antigens. This is a common consequence of pregnancy and the proportion of women who become immunized increases with increasing numbers of pregnancies.

- Patients who have had a number of transfusions of red blood cells or platelet components, may become immunized to the MHC antigens on leukocytes present in the transfusion.

- Patients who have had a previous transplant and rejected it, will almost certainly have antibodies to any foreign MHC antigens which were present on that graft.

Antibodies to major blood group antigens may also cause hyperacute rejection if they are already present in the recipient. For example, the blood group A, B and H antigens are present on the endothelial cells that line blood vessels. If a recipient of blood group A is given a transplant, such as a kidney, from a person of blood group B, the anti-B in the recipient's plasma will attack the endothelial cells of the graft, activating complement and causing destruction of the graft. Hyperacute rejection occurs rapidly and, for this reason, transplants of large organs are no longer carried out against an ABO barrier.

The fact that preformed antibodies can cause rapid rejection of a graft means that it is very important to know which potential recipients have such antibodies and, for this reason, a cross-match is performed in which serum from the recipient is incubated with cells from the donor.

Graft versus host disease (GVHD)

GVHD occurs when **both** of the following conditions are met:

- The recipient cannot reject the graft due to an underlying immune deficiency.
- The graft contains immunocompetent cells.

This is therefore a problem when carrying out an allogeneic bone marrow transplant and can be a serious limitation to bone marrow transplantation. T lymphocytes in the bone marrow respond to foreign MHC antigens on the recipient's cells and mount an immunological attack. GVHD may occur between 7 and 30 days following transfusion of small lymphocytes. In the acute form of GVHD there is an extensive skin rash which may be confused initially with an allergic reaction. The epithelial cells of the skin become necrotic and may be sloughed off. Similar occurrences in the intestine lead to diarrhoea. The liver and spleen may be affected, leading to enlargement of these organs and jaundice. Acute GVHD may result in the death of the patient. Chronic GVHD involves chronic desquamation of the skin, diarrhoea, spleen and liver enlargement and frequent secondary infections.

Transfusion-associated GVHD

It is now recognized that GVHD is a rare complication of transfusion of whole blood and blood products which contain residual leukocytes. It is particularly associated with transfusion of immunodeficient individuals (though not those with AIDS) and patients with aplastic anaemia, and may also occur following intrauterine transfusion of a foetus or transfusion of premature neonates whose immune systems are immature. GVHD has been associated with transfusion of packed red cells, platelets and fresh plasma, all of which may contain residual T lymphocytes. It is now recommended that such products be subjected to gamma irradiation (25–50 Gy) prior to transfusion to prevent any small lymphocytes from dividing. Plasma that has been frozen is safe since the freezing process (in the absence of any cryoprotective agent) destroys the leukocytes.

The major histocompatibility complex (MHC)

As mentioned above, the major histocompatibility complex is a genetic region which codes for several different types of protein, classified as Class I, Class II and Class III. Class I MHC genes code for proteins found on the surface of all nucleated cells. They are integral membrane proteins which present antigens to CD8+ T lymphocytes (see Chapter 1). Class II MHC genes also code for integral membrane proteins, but these are found on a restricted range of cells. Many of these cell types act as 'antigen-presenting cells' and present 'exogenous' antigen to CD4+ T lymphocytes.

Class III genes code for a variety of soluble proteins and are not relevant to this discussion. Examples of genes found within this region are those that code for the complement proteins C4 and C2 and the genes for different forms of tumour necrosis factor (TNF).

Class I proteins

All Class I MHC proteins have a similar overall structure, as shown in Figure 11.1. This consists of a single polypeptide chain (molecular weight 45 000 Da) known as the alpha (α) chain. It is a transmembrane protein which has three distinct immunoglobulin-like domains, α_1 α_2 and α_3. This protein is always associated in the membrane with a smaller polypeptide known as β_2 microglobulin (β_2M; molecular weight 12 000 Da). This is not a transmembrane protein and is not encoded by the MHC. It seems to be necessary for the stability of the α chain in the membrane.

Different Class I molecules are encoded at different genetic loci and these reflect fundamental differences between the overall amino acid sequences of the α chain. However, antigenic differences also occur between different forms of a Class I molecule encoded within a single genetic locus. These variations are due to allelic variations in genes at a particular locus. In this case, the differences in amino acid sequences which cause antigenic variations occur mostly in the α_1 and α_2 domains.

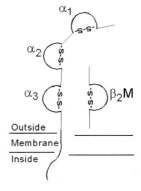

Figure 11.1 *The Class I MHC molecule consists of a single α chain encoded by the MHC. This chain is always associated in the membrane with the smaller β_2 microglobulin, which is not encoded within the MHC*

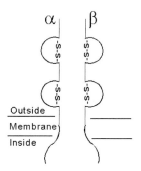

Figure 11.2 *Each Class II MHC molecule consists of two different polypeptide chains, both of which are encoded within the MHC*

Class II proteins

Class II proteins are made up of two polypeptide chains: an α chain (molecular weight 33 000 Da) and a β chain (molecular weight 28 000 Da). Both chains are encoded within the MHC. They are both transmembrane proteins with two immunoglobulin-like domains each (see Figure 11.2). There are several genetic loci encoding different Class II α and β chains within the Class II region of the MHC. In addition, there is considerable antigenic variation between Class II molecules specified at the same locus which is accounted for by allelic variation. This will be discussed below in the context of the human MHC, which is otherwise known as the **HLA system**. The antigenic variation within Class II molecules specified at an individual locus is caused by amino acid sequence variations in the α_1 and β_1 domains.

HLA stands for human leukocyte antigens. This is because they were first discovered from the observation, in 1958, that sera from patients who had received multiple blood transfusions would agglutinate leukocytes. Of course, it is now known that these antigens are not confined to leukocytes. Moreover, there are many leukocyte antigens which are not encoded by the HLA region. However, the human MHC is still universally known as the HLA system.

The HLA system

The HLA complex is found on the short arm of chromosome 6. A very simplified diagram of the HLA complex is shown in Figure 11.3. The Class I region contains several genetic loci and in each of these is a gene encoding a Class I α chain. The best known loci are HLA-A, HLA-B and HLA-C, though others have been discovered more recently. The genes at each of these loci encode a different Class I protein. These genes are isotypes, which means that the cells of the body express the products of each of these genes. In addition,

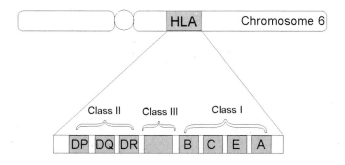

Figure 11.3 *The HLA complex is located on chromosome 6. The Class I, II and III regions are shown here*

since chromosomes come in pairs, the homologous chromosome 6 also contains the HLA-A, HLA-B and HLA-C loci. The genes within the loci on the two homologous chromosome are alleles. This means that they are alternative forms of the genes, coding for proteins with slight variations in amino acid sequence (usually in the α_1 domain). These paired genes are co-dominant, which means that both alleles are expressed in cells. Therefore, nucleated cells in the body express two slightly different HLA-A proteins in their membranes as well as two different HLA-B proteins and two different HLA-C proteins.

Polymorphisms

In classical Mendelian genetics a gene may exist in two allelic forms. These alleles have slightly different base sequences so that the proteins they encode will have similarly slight differences in amino acid composition. Depending on where these changes occur, the change of amino acid sequence may or may not affect the activity of the protein. However, even minor changes in terms of amino acid composition can affect the immunogenicity.

Within a population, there are some genes that exist in many different allelic forms although an individual within a population has only two of these alleles (one on each homologous chromosome). Such a system is said to be **polymorphic**. The MHC in higher vertebrates is one of the most highly polymorphic systems known and the HLA complex in man is no exception. So far, 108 alleles of the A gene, 223 alleles of the B gene and 67 alleles of the C gene have been discovered by sequencing the DNA encoding individual genes. Given that each individual has two of these alleles at each locus, it will be seen that the chances of individuals having the same 'set' of HLA genes is very small.

The Class II region

Within the Class II region are several genetic loci, the best known being DP, DQ and DR. Within each of these loci there are genes encoding the α and the β chains of the Class II molecules. The situation is rather more complex than for Class I, in that there may be more than one gene at each locus encoding the α and the β chains. For example, the HLA-DR region contains four genes for the HLA-β chain. All of these β-chain products may be expressed in a single cell, making the degree of variation much higher. Like Class I, the Class II region also displays a high degree of polymorphism (see Table 11.4 for details).

HLA typing

Traditionally, tissue typing has been carried out using serological methods. These use antibodies against individual HLA antigens to

---

Originally the Class II region was known as the HLA-D region and was discovered, not serologically, but by genetic differences between small lymphocytes which would allow them to stimulate each other when cultured together in a technique known as the **mixed lymphocyte reaction (MLR)**. Subsequently, anti-HLA sera were discovered which distinguished a number of proteins specified by genes at different loci within the HLA-D region.

Alleles of HLA genes have been discovered in two different ways. Originally new alleles were discovered when transplantation scientists found antisera with 'new' specificities against human lymphocytes. However, the newer techniques of DNA sequencing have allowed far more alleles to be discovered, even though no antibodies against the products of these alleles have necessarily been found. Thus the number of alleles determined serologically is far lower than the number determined by DNA sequencing methods. New alleles are confirmed at major international workshops which have met regularly since they were set up in the 1960s.

Table 11.4 *Polymorphism of Class II genes**

Gene	Codes for:	Number of alleles
HLA-DRB	β chain of HLA-DR	249
HLA-DQA1	α chain of HLA-DQ	20
HLA-DQB1	β chain of HLA-DQ	36
HLA-DPA1	α chain of HLA-DP	13
HLA-DPB1	β chain of HLA-DP	82

* The alleles so named are based on data obtained by sequencing the DNA; information has been obtained from the Internet site www.anthonynolan. com/HIG/index.html.

detect the corresponding antigens on the surface of peripheral blood lymphocytes (PBL). Today, serological methods are being used alongside molecular biology methods and the latter have been particularly useful in typing for genes within the Class II region.

Serological methods

The most usual method is the **lymphocytotoxicity assay**. PBL are used when typing for Class I antigens and these are easily obtained from fresh whole blood. When typing for Class II antigens, B lymphocytes are used since T lymphocytes do not express Class II molecules. B lymphocytes can be obtained by enrichment from PBL by one of several methods.

For the lymphocytotoxicity assay, aliquots of freshly isolated, viable PBL or enriched B lymphocytes are pipetted into the wells of a 96-well microcytotoxicity plate (known as a Teresaki plate). Antibodies to individual HLA antigens are added to individual wells. An antibody will bind to a small lymphocyte if the appropriate antigen is present on these cells. When complement is added, the cells are killed owing to activation of the classical pathway (see Chapter 3). Viability stains, which only stain dead cells, are added to each well and thus those wells in which an antibody has bound to an antigen will be seen to contain dead cells.

Cross-matching

This is a test to detect preformed antibodies to graft antigens in the serum of a potential recipient. The test can be performed in a lymphocytotoxicity assay in which serum from the recipient is incubated with PBL from the donor. Complement is added and the viability of the cells tested as previously described. If donor cells are killed it indicates that the recipient already has antibodies against graft antigens and is likely to be an unsuitable match.

Anti-HLA antibodies are usually obtained from the sera of multiparous women. The specificity of these antibodies is first determined by screening them in a lymphocytotoxicity assay against a panel of cells of known HLA types. For Class II typing, B lymphocytes are incubated with antisera to individual Class II antigens. Since most anti-HLA sera also contain antibodies to Class I antigens, these must be removed from the antiserum by incubating with pooled platelets which also express Class I antigens. The platelets 'absorb' the anti-Class I antibodies and are removed by centrifugation.

Rabbit serum is used as a source of complement. Trypan blue and eosin-Y are suitable viable stains. An alternative method is to stain the small lymphocytes with a fluorescent dye prior to testing. When the cells are killed the dye leaks out and the cells are no longer visible under a fluorescence microscope. A test is scored as strongly positive when more than 50% of the cells in a well are killed.

Molecular biology techniques

Techniques based on the detection of DNA coding for an antigen, rather than serological methods which detect the antigen itself, are currently being used to type for Class II antigens. Two such techniques are described below.

Restriction fragment length polymorphisms (RFLPs)

The basis for this test is that DNA which varies in base sequence will produce different sized fragments of DNA when 'cut' by restriction enzymes (bacterial endonucleases which cut DNA at specific base sequences). The fragments can be separated out by size using gel electrophoresis and transferred onto nylon membranes by blotting. The nylon membranes are then incubated with labelled DNA probes complementary to certain consensus sequences. This procedure will produce a banding pattern characteristic of certain alleles. This method requires a relatively large amount of DNA (between 5 and 10 ug).

Polymerase chain reaction (PCR)

PCR is used to amplify an area of DNA by using primers specific for that particular region and the enzyme DNA polymerase. The method rapidly allows the production of multiple copies of a targeted area of DNA. The amplified portions of HLA genes may be analysed by electrophoresis, blotting and probing with short oligonucleotide probes which hybridize to sequences characteristic of particular HLA Class II alleles. PCR methods are useful because they require much less DNA initially. They can also be carried out on whole blood that has been stored frozen without a cryoprotective agent because, unlike serological assays, they do not require the presence of live cells.

Bone marrow transplantation

Bone marrow is a source of haemopoietic stem cells. These cells are the early progenitors of all the mature cellular elements in the blood: the red cells, the white cells and the platelets. In the bone marrow these cells are constantly dividing. Their progeny are capable of giving rise to any of the cells in the blood, i.e. they are **totipotent**. The technique of transplanting haemopoietic stem cells is of value in the treatment of various malignant disorders, particularly leukaemia, and for disorders in which the normal production of healthy blood cells by the bone marrow has been affected by infection, malignant changes or inherited disorders. This may involve total bone marrow failure, such as in aplastic anaemia, or partial failure, as seen in a range of haemoglobinopathies. Another indication for bone marrow transplant is in cases where there are deficiencies of enzyme production, such as inborn errors of metabolism. A bone marrow transplant provides a source of stem cells, which migrate to the marrow of the patient and continue to produce immature blood cells, thus restoring normal haemopoiesis. The laboratory techniques involved in bone marrow transplantation have now become standard in many blood centres and hospital transfusion departments.

Availability and choice of donors

Donors of bone marrow for transplant are preferably related to the patient as this decreases the chance of GVHD. However, compatible related donors are available in only about 30% of cases and, increasingly, unrelated donors are used. Currently, in the UK, the details of approximately four million volunteer donors are kept by the donor bone marrow panels. The development of tissue typing using molecular techniques has reduced the risk of GVHD in bone marrow transplant recipients.

Factors affecting compatibility

The major difficulty in achieving a successful allogeneic bone marrow transplant comes from differences in the HLA system between donor and recipient. Differences in Class II HLA antigens are particularly relevant here. Problems of compatibility are increased when the bone marrow transplant donor is unrelated to the patient requiring the transplant. The severity of GVHD is directly related to the degree of incompatibility, especially in the Class II region, and many patients do not have an HLA-identical sibling. In these circumstances, a combination of techniques is used at a serological, cellular and molecular level in an attempt to provide the most compatible transplant.

If a bone marrow transplant is the treatment strategy of choice, the initial approach is to HLA type the parents and siblings of the patient. Sometimes an identical HLA donor is found and in other cases a partial HLA mismatched relative may be an option. In mismatched donors it is even more important to HLA type thoroughly, and again cellular and molecular techniques improve the likelihood of successful matching.

Techniques for haemopoietic stem cell collection and transplant

Allogeneic bone marrow transplant

The marrow is harvested from various sites, particularly from both iliac crests of the hip bone, whilst the donor is under general anaesthesia. The aim is to collect sufficient cells to ensure speedy engraftment – usually a minimum of 3×10^8 nucleated bone

CD34 is a cell surface antigen which is expressed on human and mouse haemopoietic stem cells – both **totipotent cells** which have the capacity to develop into any line of blood cell, and **lineage-committed progenitor cells** which, as their name suggests, are committed to develop into a specific cell type. They account for approximately 1% of bone marrow cells and are rarely found in peripheral blood. The structure of CD34 consists of a core protein backbone which is highly glycosylated and includes sialic acid residues. Experiments using *in vivo* transgenesis have shown that CD34 promotes adhesion to bone marrow stroma. The CD34 gene has been investigated to further our knowledge of the involvement of CD34 in haemopoiesis.

marrow cells per kilogram of recipient body weight. This cell number contains approximately 2×10^6 **CD34+**, cells per kilogram of recipient body weight.

At this stage the marrow may be infused into the recipient or it may require further processing. If there is a difference in ABO blood group between the donor and recipient it is necessary to further treat the marrow to remove the red cells or contaminating plasma. Techniques are also available to remove T cells from the graft which can reduce both the incidence and severity of GVHD. One method that may be used is to incubate the bone marrow cells with an antibody to CD3, a protein which is present on the membranes of all mature T lymphocytes. Addition of complement results in the lysis of these T cells.

Bone marrow stem cells are transfused into the patient intravenously and progress is then monitored and transfusion support therapy given.

Autologous bone marrow transplant

Using an autologous bone marrow transplant (i.e. from the same individual) prevents the occurrence of GVHD completely, although it has been shown to be less successful in preventing recurrence of malignant disease. For an autologous bone marrow transplant, marrow is harvested from the patient whilst in remission from the disease due to treatment. This negates the need for a compatible donor. However, where the transplant is used to treat a malignancy such as leukaemia, it is necessary to 'purge' the marrow of any malignant cells whilst preserving the viable haemopoietic stem cells. Several techniques, based on the physical, pharmacological or immunological properties of the contaminating malignant cells, are available.

Peripheral blood stem cell transplantation

Until 1986 the major source of stem cells was bone marrow. More recently, peripheral blood stem cell transplantation (PBSCT) has largely replaced bone marrow as a source of autologous haemopoietic blood cells and there have been significant advances in the use of allogeneic PBSCT. However, stem cells are rarely found in the circulation and, in order to increase the number of circulating stem cells for harvesting, the cells must be 'mobilized' from the marrow into the peripheral blood by injection of granulocyte-colony stimulating factor (G-CSF). This cytokine acts, as the name suggests, to stimulate the production of haemopoietic cells, and in particular those cells which express the cell surface antigen CD34.

Reasons for the popularity of PBSCT include the ease of collection using the technique of **apheresis** and the reduced likelihood of the graft being affected by the presence of tumour cells from existing disease. In addition, higher numbers of CD34+ cells can often be obtained and this is reflected in an improved time to engraftment. It is now possible to isolate CD34+ cells to high levels of purity, thus significantly reducing the number of unwanted cells (see Figure 11.4).

Human umbilical cord blood

A further rich source of haemopoietic stem cells is umbilical cord blood. The success of umbilical cord blood transplantation in matched siblings has led to the establishment of cord blood banks in an attempt to further increase the unrelated donor pool. Umbilical cord blood is harvested with maternal consent, HLA typed and cryopreserved until required. The early results for unrelated cord blood look promising but the value of this technique is still being investigated.

Storage of transplant material

Patients requiring a bone marrow transplant may be given immunosuppressive treatment prior to the procedure in an attempt to prevent graft rejection, depending on the reasons for transplantation. This is achieved by a combination of irradiation and/or cytotoxic drugs and may form part of the treatment for a malignant disease. It may therefore be necessary to store the harvested stem cells prior to infusion. Short-term (between 2 and 3 days) storage of bone marrow should be within a blood transfusion refrigerator at 4°C and PBSC should be stored at 21–22°C with agitation to prevent platelet aggregation. Longer-term storage requires cryopreservation in a programmed rate freezer with 10% dimethyl sulphoxide as a cryoprotective agent. Storage is then in the gas or liquid phase of liquid nitrogen (approximately −70°C).

Transfusion support post-transplant

Blood components such as red blood cells and platelets are needed for support therapy of a post-transplant patient. It is necessary to irradiate these components with γ rays as the process of irradiation prevents contaminating lymphocytes being activated. Many laboratories possess a blood irradiator and it is a simple process to place the blood component inside, usually for 2 minutes. Another important consideration is the provision of blood components that are known to be negative for cytomegalovirus (CMV). This is because the immunosuppressed patient will be prone to infection from a variety of sources, including blood components. The transfusion of CMV positive blood components may cause a recurrence of earlier CMV infection that has remained dormant in the patient.

Apheresis is a technique that is used for collection of specific blood components and has the advantage that blood is returned to the donor. This allows donations to be taken more frequently. In the collection of peripheral blood stem cells, a series of apheresis sessions take place over a few hours with minimum discomfort to the donor. Apheresis is also used for collection of blood components (see Chapter 7).

The International Bone Marrow Transplant Registry (IBMTR) and the Autologous Blood and Marrow Registry (ABMTR) are international research organizations that collect data on haemopoietic stem cell transplant recipients worldwide. The resulting databases have information on more than 65 000 transplant recipients, representing approximately 40% of allogeneic transplants since 1964 and 50% of autologous transplants performed in America since 1989. Follow-up of patients and analysis of data provide the means to assess the most appropriate treatment.

Figure 11.4 *Scattergrams showing CD34 analysis of peripheral blood stem cells using flow cytometry. The vertical axis indicates side-scatter and the horizontal axis indicates fluorescence intensity. Stem cells are characterized by low scatter. (a) Pre-selection: CD34+ cells make up 0.7% of the population. (b) Post-selection: CD34+ cells make up 96% of the population. The CD34+ cells have been selected using magnetic activated cell sorting. (Courtesy of T.F. Carr, Royal Manchester Children's Hospital, Salford, UK)*

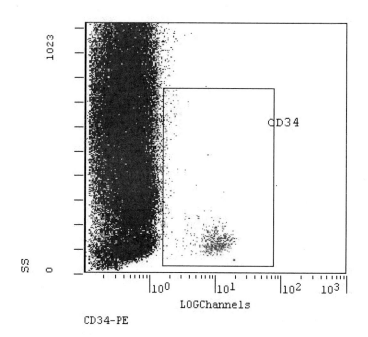

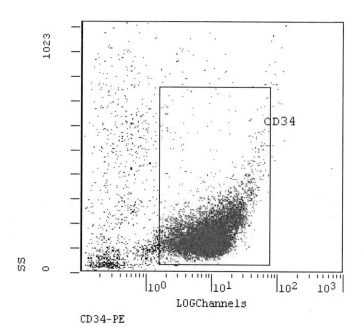

Suggested further reading

Colombe, B.W. (1994). Histocompatibility testing. In *Basic and Clinical Immunology* (eds D.P. Stites, A.I. Terr and T.G. Parslow). Oxford: Stamford.

Dyer, P. and Middleton, D., eds (1993). *Histocompatibility Testing: A Practical Approach*. Oxford: IRL Press.

Horowitz, M.M. and Rowlings, P.A. (1997). An update from the International Bone Marrow Transplant Registry on current activity in haemopoietic stem cell transplantation. *Current Opinion in Hematology*, **4**, 395–400.

Link, H. and Arseniev, L. (1997). CD34+ blood cells for allogeneic progenitor and stem cell transplantation. *Leukaemia and Lymphoma*, **26**, 451–465.

Page, G. and Paul, N. (1995). An introduction to tissue typing: Internet site http://www.umds.ac.uk/tissue/.

Self-assessment questions

1. Outline the difference between an autograft and an allograft (allogeneic graft).
2. What is meant by a 'histocompatibility antigen'?
3. State what feature of the immune system is responsible for:
   (a) hyperacute rejection of a transplant;
   (b) acute rejection of a transplant.
4. When may a blood transfusion cause graft versus host disease?
5. How do Class I and Class II MHC molecules differ in their tissue distribution?
6. How are tissues 'typed'?
7. List some disorders in which stem cell transplantation has been of value.
8. Define the cells on which CD34 antigen is expressed.
9. List the benefits of umbilical cord blood stem cells compared to other options.
10. Give examples of problems concerning post-transfusion support in stem cell transplant patients.

Key Concepts and Facts

- Transplantation of a wide variety of organs and tissues is now a common and successful occurrence.

- Rejection of transplants may be mediated by preformed antibody (hyperacute) or by T cells (acute).

- Successful bone marrow or stem cell transplants have cured many previously incurable diseases such as leukaemia.

- Success in transplantation depends on histocompatibility between the donor and recipient in order to prevent graft rejection or the development of graft versus host disease.

- The histocompatibility antigens of most importance are those encoded by the HLA region, which is the human MHC. This system is highly polymorphic.

- Tissue typing can be carried out with a mixture of serological and molecular techniques, the latter being of increasing importance in bone marrow and stem cell transplantation.

- Sources of stem cells include peripheral blood and umbilical cord blood in addition to bone marrow.

Answers to self-assessment questions

Chapter 1

1. The two work very closely together: products of specific immunity affect the non-specific responses and *vice versa*.
2. Specificity and immunological memory.
3. They are secreted by cells and they affect other cells by binding to cell surface receptors and stimulating transmembrane events.
4. Neutrophils – blood; monocytes – blood; macrophages – found throughout the body. Collectively phagocytes are found everywhere and this is important because foreign material can enter at any site in the body.
5. The process brings plasma and neutrophils into an area of tissue damage in which infection might occur.
6. When it is prolonged, for example, by a chronic infection.
7. On the whole, humoral immunity deals with extracellular pathogens while cell-mediated immunity deals with intracellular pathogens.
8. A bacterium is made up of many different proteins, glycoproteins, lipoproteins etc., each of which is immunogenic.
9. From the bursa of Fabricius where they develop in birds.
10. They all have different cell surface receptors for an epitope.
11. In specific immunity, small lymphocytes exposed to an immunogen first proliferate before they differentiate. Specific immunity depends on cell division.

Chapter 2

1. (a) IgG; (b) IgM; (c) IgE; (d) IgA.
2. Immunoglobulins are classified according to the type of heavy chain they possess.
3. IgG is used for passive immunization because it has a relatively long half-life.
4. IgM has μ heavy chains whereas IgG has γ heavy chains. IgM is a pentameric structure whereas IgG is monomeric.
5. The variable regions of heavy chains of immunoglobulins from different plasma cells always have a different amino acid

sequence. The sequence of amino acids in all antibodies of the same class remains the same in the constant region.

6. Any two of: to activate complement; to control transfer across the placenta; to activate phagocytes; to bind to large granular lymphocytes.

7. Any three of: steric; hydrophobic; hydrogen bonds; ionic interaction; van der Waals forces.

8. Affinity describes the strength of binding of a single binding site for an epitope. Avidity describes the strength of binding of antibodies to an immunogen.

9. By binding to receptors for IgG on phagocytes and stimulating phagocytosis; by activating complement – some complement proteins opsonize immunogens, others attract neutrophils and some stimulate inflammation.

Chapter 3

1. IgM is the most efficient antibody at stimulating haemolysis.

2. The activation of complement involves a number of enzymic stages which cause amplification in the system.

3. Newly activated complement proteins often have a transient hydrophobic binding site which allows them to bind to the cell membrane of the antibody-coated cell.

4. An anaphylatoxin stimulates degranulation of mast cells and basophils. The histamine released causes vasodilation and inflammation. Chemotactic factors for neutrophils and eosinophils attract these cells into the site of complement activation.

5. Complement levels may be assessed by looking at the ability of the serum to lyse sheep red cells coated with sub-agglutinating levels of antibody.

6. Complement may be inactivated by heating to 56°C for 30 minutes. Calcium and magnesium ions are needed for complement activation. EDTA is a chelating agent and effectively removes these ions from a solution to which it is added.

Chapter 4

1. A codon is a triplet of bases, for example adenine, guanine and cytosine, which codes for a specific amino acid or acts as a stop/start signal.

2. An allele refers to a gene which exists in alternative forms at the same locus of homologous chromosomes.

3. The DNA organic bases are adenine, guanine, cytosine and thymine.

4. Inheritance via autosomal chromosomes.

5. Independent assortment takes place during the separation of chromatids in meiosis. It occurs when genes of homologous chromosomes are situated too far apart to be inherited

together, or in genes of non-homologous chromosomes. Dependent assortment occurs in genes on the same chromosome where the loci, i.e. positions on the chromosome, are close. Thus the genes move together to the newly formed sex cells during the process of 'crossing over' of chromatids in meiosis.

6. The role of tRNA is to transfer amino acids from the cell pool to the ribosomes where they attach to the opposite base pairs of the codon in mRNA, thus forming a polypeptide chain.

7. Three types of mutation are: silent mutation, when an amino acid is substituted for another but it has no evident effect on the phenotype; mis-sense mutation, when substitutions of bases result in a change in the amino acid sequence which may then result in the formation of an abnormal protein; and frame-shift mutations due to insertion or deletion of bases which cause changes in the codon, resulting in a change to the reading frame.

Chapter 5

1. A gene: encodes for production of N-acetyl-galactosaminyl transferase. B gene: encodes for production of D-galactosyl transferase. H gene: encodes for production of L-fucose. Se gene: encodes for production of (2-L-fucosyl transferase. Z gene: regulates production of the H antigen on red cells. O gene: encodes for production of inactive polypeptide chain.

2. ABH red cell antigens are oligosaccharides present on glycoproteins and glycolipids that are attached to the red cell membrane. ABH substances are glycoproteins; the sugar molecules are attached by type 1 and type 2 linkages. The secretor gene is required for the substances to be secreted from endodermically derived cells.

3. Caucasians are predominantly group A or O; group B is less common and AB is rare. Group O is also most common in Blacks but there is a higher percentage of group B people, roughly equivalent to group A. By contrast, group B is most common in the Indian population.

4. Two loci exist: the *RHD* gene which forms the RHD polypeptide expressing the D antigen, and the *RHCE* gene which forms the RHCE polypeptide expressing the C/c and E/e antigens.

5. The five major antigens of the Rh system are: D, C, c, E and e.

6. Rh immune antibodies attach to red cells at 37°C. The antiglobulin test or enzyme-treated red cells are used for their detection.

Chapter 6

1. Le^a, Le^b, P_1, P^k, I, and i. Also, A, B and H antigens are carbohydrate structures.
2. Antigens that are protein structures are MNSs, Lutheran, Kell, Duffy, Kidd and Rh antigens.
3. I and i antigens differ in that I is a branched carbohydrate series and i is a linear carbohydrate structure. Furthermore, I is expressed on adult red cells whilst i is expressed on infants' red cells. The i antigen is converted to the branched form by an enzyme as the individual matures.
4. Complement-binding antibodies include: P system antibodies; anti-I; antibodies of the Duffy and Kidd systems; and some antibodies of Le^a and Le^b blood groups.
5. Glycophorin A of the MN system acts as a receptor for *P. falciparum*; also Duffy antigens form the site of attachment for *P. vivax*.

Chapter 7

1. Warm haemolytic anaemia is caused by antibodies which cause haemolysis of red cells at 37°C, i.e. body temperature. These antibodies may be connected with viral infections, tumours or immune diseases such as SLE.
2. Cold haemolytic anaemia occurs when antibodies are produced which attach to red cells at lower temperatures, from approximately 4 to 28°C. They may arise in response to infection (e.g. with *M. pneumoniae* or Epstein–Barr virus).
3. Free haemoglobin may be detected in the plasma or in the urine. The breakdown of haemoglobin results in raised levels of bilirubin in the circulation.
4. There are three types of drug-induced haemolytic anaemia: (a) That where antibodies induced due to the presence of the drug form a complex with the drug and attach to the red cells. (b) That involving membrane modification, where antibodies are formed due to proteins on the red cell surface which are induced by the presence of the drug. (c) That where antibodies are formed in response to the attachment of the drug on to the surface of the red cells.
5. Kernicterus refers to the accumulation of bilirubin in the brain. This results in damaged brain tissue. The levels of bilirubin may be reduced either by phototherapy with ultraviolet light, or by exchange transfusion of blood.
6. Anti-D immunoglobulin should be given to all Rh negative pregnant women, either within 72 hours of childbirth or after any adverse event resulting in loss of the foetus, or post amniocentesis or other trauma that may have caused leakage of foetal cells into the mother.
7. The Kleihauer–Betke stain is based on the principle that foetal

haemoglobin is resistant to elution from the red cells in an acid environment whereas adult (maternal) haemoglobin is not. This results in pink foetal cells which may be counted to estimate the number present in the mother's circulation.

Chapter 8

1. Red cell concentrate, platelets, fresh frozen plasma, cryoprecipitate.
2. Massive blood loss (together with a volume expander), anaemia, pre- and post-surgery, during surgery.
3. Platelets should be stored at room temperature and constantly agitated.
4. 2,3-DPG lowers the affinity of haemoglobin for oxygen so that the oxygen is released to the tissues.
5. Leukocytes are viral transmitters, especially of cytomegalovirus; they present the antigens of the HLA system; they produce cytokines.
6. Irradiation, which inactivates virus-carrying leukocytes, or filtering, which removes them; heat treatment to 80°C for 72 hours; use of chemicals.

Chapter 9

1. Temperature, pH, ionic strength, antigen and antibody concentration.
2. (a) Inadequate washing of the red cells prior to the addition of AHG regent. (b) Faulty reading technique leading to disruption of agglutinates.
3. (a) The enzymes remove negative surface charge from the red cell by removing glycophorins. This reduction in charge allows the red cells to approach one another more closely, so that the small IgG antibodies can span the gap between adjacent red cells. (b) By removing proteins from the red cell surface, enzymes may make hidden antigen sites more accessible to antibody. (c) Similarly they may increase the mobility of proteins within the membrane, allowing for antigen clustering and the formation of multiple intercellular bridges. (d) Enzymes reduce hydration at the red cell surface which favours antigen/antibody binding. (e) They promote the formation of irregular protrusions from the red cells. These protrusions exhibit less repulsive force due to their highly curved surfaces.
4. Ionic bonds, hydrogen bonds, hydrophobic bonds, van der Waals forces or randomization of water.
5. Due to the electrical charges involved, on the red cells and in the saline, the zeta potential keeps the red cells apart by a minimum distance of approximately 20 nm. IgM antibodies

have a distance between binding sites of approximately 30 nm and so can bridge the gap between adjacent red cells. The binding sites of IgG antibodies are only approximately 12 nm apart and so cannot bridge the gap between red cells suspended in saline.

Chapter 10

1. HIV, HBV, HCV and syphilis.
2. Clerical error at the time of sample collection from the patient, collection of donor blood from the laboratory or at the time of transfusion – leading to transfusion of the blood to the wrong patient.
3. Febrile and urticarial reactions due to anti-white cell antibodies, cytokines or allergens.
4. All reactions should be reported to the hospital transfusion laboratory in the first instance. Then, bacterial or viral infections should be reported to the local transfusion centre. Adverse reactions to plasma fractions are reported to the Committee for the Safety of Medicines. Haemolytic and anaphylactic reactions resulting from the transfusion of blood components are reported to the Serious Hazards of Transfusion group.
5. By gamma irradiation of the red cell or platelet component to inactivate the donor's white cells.
6. Iron overload.
7. Post-transfusion purpura may occur as a result of anti-platelet antibodies in the patient which destroy the transfused donor platelets, or may be due to sequestration of the patient's platelets in the spleen in association with transfused micro-aggregates.
8. The risks of viral transmission may be minimized by careful selection of donors, testing of donors and inactivation of viruses in plasma fractions by heat or chemical treatment of the product.
9. The patient's post-transfusion sample should be tested for ABO and Rh D type. It should be screened for clinically significant red cell antibodies. A direct antiglobulin test should be performed and the sample cross-matched again against all available donor units (used and unused).

Chapter 11

1. An autograft is transferred within an individual. An allograft is transferred between two individuals.
2. A histocompatibility antigen is a cell surface protein which stimulates rejection of a graft.
3. (a) Antibodies; (b) T lymphocytes.

4. When it contains viable lymphocytes and is given to an immunodeficient individual or a premature neonate.

5. Class I molecules are found on all nucleated cells. Class II molecules are restricted to antigen-presenting cells.

6. (a) Serologically, using anti-HLA antibodies. (b) By RFLP or PCR, using oligonucleotide probes.

7. Leukaemia and some other malignancies, aplastic anaemia, congenital immunodeficiency, some inherited enzyme deficiency disorders.

8. Totipotent and lineage-committed stem cells.

9. Freely available (subject to maternal permission); the process does not require cytokine treatment (as for PBSCT) or an operation (as for bone marrow).

10. Blood and blood product transfusions must be irradiated to prevent transfusion of viable lymphocytes and the development of GVHD. Blood and products should be negative for cytomegalovirus, even if the patient is already CMV positive.

Index